KEY TOPICS IN
PAIN MEDICINE
THIRD EDITION

Kate Grady
BSc MB BS FRCA
Consultant in Anaesthesia and Pain Medicine
South Manchester University Hospitals NHS Trust
Manchester, UK

Andrew Severn
MA MB FRCA
Consultant in Anaesthesia and Pain Medicine
University Hospitals of Morecambe Bay NHS Trust
Lancaster, UK

Paul Eldridge
MA MChir FRCS
Consultant Neurosurgeon
Walton Centre for Neurology and Neurosurgery
Liverpool, UK

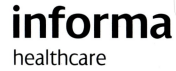
informa
healthcare

© 1997, 2002, 2007 Informa UK Ltd

First published in the United Kingdom in 1997 by BIOS

Second Edition published in 2002 by BIOS, an imprint of the Taylor & Francis Group. Taylor & Francis Group is the Academic Division of Informa plc

Third Edition published in 2007 by Informa Healthcare, 4 Park Square, Milton Park, Abingdon, Oxon OX14 4RN. Informa Healthcare is a trading division of Informa UK Ltd. Registered Office: 37/41 Mortimer Street, London W1T 3JH. Registered in England and Wales Number 1072954.

Tel: +44 (0)20 7017 6000
Fax: +44 (0)20 7017 6699
E-mail: info.medicine@tandf.co.uk
Website: www.tandf.co.uk/medicine

Although every effort has been made to ensure that all owners of copyright material have been acknowledged in this publication, we would be glad to acknowledge in subsequent reprints or editions any omissions brought to our attention.

Although every effort has been made to ensure that drug doses and other information are presented accurately in this publication, the ultimate responsibility rests with the prescribing physician. Neither the publishers nor the authors can be held responsible for errors or for any consequences arising from the use of information contained herein. For detailed prescribing information or instructions on the use of any product or procedure discussed herein, please consult the prescribing information or instructional material issued by the manufacturer.

A CIP record for this book is available from the British Library.

Library of Congress Cataloging-in-Publication Data

Data available on application

ISBN-10: 0 415 38620 9
ISBN-13: 978 0 415 38620 3

Distributed in North and South America by
Taylor & Francis
6000 Broken Sound Parkway, NW, (Suite 300)
Boca Raton, FL 33487, USA

Within Continental USA
Tel: 1 (800) 272 7737; Fax: 1 (800) 374 3401
Outside Continental USA
Tel: (561) 994 0555; Fax: (561) 361 6018
Email: orders@crcpress.com

Distributed in the rest of the world by
Thomson Publishing Services
Cheriton House
North Way
Andover, Hampshire SP10 5BE, UK
Tel: +44 (0)1264 332424
Email: tps.tandfsalesorder@thomson.com

Composition by Scribe Design Ltd, Ashford, Kent
Printed and bound in India by Replika Press Pvt Ltd

CONTENTS

[a]Includes contribution from Dr Joshua Adedokun, Specialist Registrar, North Western Rotation in Anaesthesia, UK.

[b]Contributed by Professor Andrew Smith, The Institute of Health, Lancaster University, UK.

[c]Includes contribution from Dr Barrie Tait, Avenue Consulting, Christchurch, New Zealand.

[d]Includes contribution from Dr Varun Jaitly, Consultant Anaesthetist, Wrightington, Wigan and Leigh Hospitals NHS Trust, UK.

[e]Includes contribution from Dr Radhika Bhishma, Consultant Anaesthetist, Pennine Acute Hospitals NHS Trust, UK.

[f]Includes contribution from Dr Graham Johnson, Consultant Anaesthetist, Blackpool Victoria Hospital NHS Trust, UK.

[g]Includes contribution from Dr Paul Cook, Consultant Anaesthetist, Pennine Acute Hospitals NHS Trust, UK.

[h]Contributed by Dr Barry Miller, Consultant Anaesthetist, Bolton Hospitals NHS Trust, UK.

[i]Includes contribution from Dr Barry Miller, Consultant Anaesthetist, Bolton Hospitals NHS Trust, UK.

[j]Includes contributions from Dr Richard Makin, Consultant Anaesthetist, Salford Royal Hospitals NHS Trust, UK.
and
Dr Barrie Tait, Avenue Consulting, Christchurch, New Zealand.

ABBREVIATIONS

AIDS	acquired immune deficiency syndrome
AVM	arteriovenous malformation
CABG	coronary artery bypass graft
CGRP	calcitonin gene-related peptide
CNS	central nervous system
COXIBs	cyclo-oxygenase type 2 inhibitors
CPH	chronic paroxysmal hemicrania
CPPWOP	chronic pelvic pain without obvious pathology
CPSP	central post-stroke pain
CRPS	complex regional pain syndromes
CSF	cerebrospinal fluid
CT	computed tomography
DMARDs	disease-modifying antirheumatic drugs
DREZ	dorsal root entry zone
DSM	Diagnostic and Statistical Manual
EBM	evidence-based medicine
ENT	ear, nose and throat
ESR	erythrocyte sedimentation rate
fMRI	functional magnetic resonance imaging
GABA	γ-amino butyric acid
HAD	hospital anxiety and depression index
HRT	hormone replacement therapy
IASP	International Association for the Study of Pain
IBS	irritable bowel syndrome
ICD	International Classification of Disease
LLLT	low-level laser therapy
MRI	magnetic resonance imaging
MS	multiple sclerosis
MVD	microvascular decompression
NGF	nerve growth factor
NMDA	N-methyl-D-aspartic acid
NNH	number needed to harm
NNT	number needed to treat
NSAIDs	nonsteroidal anti-inflammatory drugs
PHN	post-herpetic neuralgia
PVD	peripheral vascular disease
RCT	randomized controlled trial
SIP	sympathetically independent pain
SLR	straight leg raise
SMP	sympathetically maintained pain
SSRI	selective serotonin reuptake inhibitor
SUNCT	short-lived unilateral neuralgiform pain with conjunctival tearing
TCAA	tricyclic antidepressants

TENS	transcutaneous electrical nerve stimulation
TGN	trigeminal neuralgia
THC	tetrahydrocannabinol
TMJ	temporomandibular joint
TMJD	temporomandibular joint dysfunction
VSCC	voltage-sensitive calcium channels
WHO	World Health Organization

PREFACE TO THE THIRD EDITION

Work over the past thirty years has rejected the model of a pain mechanism as caused by a fixed rigid modality dedicated mechanism. The process, which produces pain, is plastic and changes sequentially with time. That essential mobility of mechanism exists in damaged tissue, in the peripheral nerves and spinal cord. This movement of pathology from periphery to centre proceeds with the triggering of reactive processes in the brain. It presents the therapist with a migrating distributed target.

Professor Patrick Wall

Opioids are our most powerful analgesics, but politics, prejudice and our continuing ignorance still impede optimum prescribing. What happens when opioids are given to someone in pain is different from what happens when they are given to someone not in pain. The medical use of opioids does not create drug addicts, and restrictions on this medical use hurt patients.

Professor Henry McQuay

The statements above are two of the more challenging statements about the nature of pain and its management. They support the existence of a specialty of pain medicine, with professionals from all backgrounds integrating their skills. This book attempts to describe the remit of the specialty of pain medicine. It attempts to visit some of the aspects of acute pain medicine where they can be related to chronic pain medicine; however, it is not a textbook of anaesthesia, and fuller accounts of pharmacology and specific techniques of perioperative and postoperative care will have to be sought elsewhere. Similarly, it is not a textbook of rheumatology or orthopaedics, and discussion of diagnosis and management of specific diseases is covered only to give the reader a feel for the place of pain management techniques within the overall management of these conditions.

The issue of whether acute and chronic pain medicine can be tackled in one small volume without detriment to either subject has been a challenge for the authors and reflects the wider debate in the professions as to whether the subjects should be practised and taught in a 'seamless' way. In the United Kingdom, the Royal College of Anaesthetists has established a Faculty of Pain Medicine to train medically qualified anaesthetists in the management of acute, chronic and cancer pain. Other professional groups may tend to concentrate on one or other field of practice. There is common ground: the value of opioids in treating all pain, and the possible role of acute pain management in preventing the development of chronic pain are examples of this. In other ways the subjects differ from the humane management of physiological disturbance, to a complex rehabilitation exercise.

There have been a few changes in the 4 years since the second edition was published that we need to note. The virtual eclipse of the cyclo-oxygenase type 2 inhibitors, the development of new ways of administration of opioids and the advent of new imaging technology of the brain are just a few examples. The clinical governance agenda in the United Kingdom has resulted in the publication of a number of monographs from professional groups about the management of specific conditions and the use of certain techniques: we have referred to these where appropriate. We have attempted to present the evidence to support a particular treatment: as before, we have made specific reference to systematic reviews, while recognizing that useful treatments may also be supported by less robust evidence. The clauses 'it is shown that' or 'it is reported that' refer in the text to higher and lower levels of evidence, respectively.

This third edition came out of a discussion with colleagues about a syllabus for postgraduate anaesthesia training, but we believe that it will be valuable to anyone interested in the management of pain. We have invited guest contributions from several of these colleagues, and we value their enthusiasm and commitment to the subject. Otherwise, we retain the skill and wisdom of the guest authors Andrew Smith and Barrie Tait from the previous edition, together with helpful comments from those whom we acknowledged last time.

PREFACE TO THE SECOND EDITION

Four years after the publication of *Key Topics in Chronic Pain* it is time to ask what has changed. When we considered the invitation, the opportunity to modernize a few chapters was tempting, but we did not anticipate a complete revision.

The science of evidence-based medicine is evolving. Four years ago a few systematic reviews were easy to acquire, and relevant randomized controlled trials could be numbered. Now there are hundreds of each and we have had to be selective in choosing those which we believe are relevant to practice. We have therefore removed many references to randomized controlled trials in favour of systematic reviews. We have asked an expert to steer us through the conflicting principles of evidence-based medicine to allow us to publish treatments according to the quality of evidence afforded. At the same time we have kept an ear out for the respected colleagues who have valuable advice to offer on managing difficult problems. We have used the term 'it is reported that' or 'it is claimed that' for anecdotal, case report and uncontrolled observations, and the term 'it is shown that' or 'it is proven' for controlled trials. The last edition was designed specifically for the needs of postgraduate trainees in anaesthesia. This edition, we hope, will introduce the subject in a real way to other doctors, of all specialties and grades, and to nurses, therapists, psychologists and alternative practitioners.

The management of chronic pain is the science and art of rehabilitation. We believe that this concept sets apart legitimate approaches, by whomever they are practised, from less valuable treatments. There is pressure from all sides to respect opinions from a variety of sources, both 'conventional' and 'alternative'. It is not the function of this book to judge the various contenders for a rightful place in multidisciplinary practice, but it can at least set some rules by which practice can be judged.

Chronic pain remains a growing subspecialty, and its coexistence with the discipline of acute pain management is a relationship we are keen to promote. Hence the reader will find chapters on burn pain and pain during pregnancy, in the hope that a handy reference to taxing 'acute pain' problems will be available here.

The relationship between doctors, managers and their political masters has changed irrevocably in four years, and we have therefore made reference to this and the relationship of the pain clinician to the local community. By strange coincidence the day the manuscript was delivered to the publishers was also the day that Professor Patrick Wall died (8th of August 2001). Patrick Wall was a major influence on the philosophy of this book. His seminal 1965 paper with Ronald Melzack which described the 'gate control' theory of pain is an example of his influence. His direct personal encouragement of one of the authors and the opinions which he so eloquently expressed at scientific meetings and which have found their way into the text is another. We hope that in some measure through the text the spirit of Patrick Wall's challenging approach to the problems of patients with pain will be passed on to another generation of clinicians.

Our trainees have been at the forefront of our minds when writing this, and we are pleased to see many moving on to consultant posts around the world. We could not have started without the encouragement of Sara and Frank, and are privileged to welcome Paul Eldridge, a neurosurgeon, as an author. Andrew Smith, who is Editor of the Cochrane Anaesthesia Review Group, and Barrie Tait, a rehabilitation specialist, have contributed to the text. We also acknowledge the support of Jai Kulkarni, Michael Sharpe, Wendy Makin and Charles Cox for commenting on the manuscripts and Chris Glynn for his help in pulling the project together.

PREFACE TO THE FIRST EDITION

This latest volume in the Key Topics series aims to provide the health professional with up-to-date information about a range of issues in the management of chronic pain. It is not a substitute for the larger texts, nor is it an attempt to provide a comprehensive reference to palliative care or painful rheumatological and neurological conditions. It is a working manual of the common problems of management of the chronic pain sufferer, the patient in whom investigations have excluded treatable disease. The book is designed for specialist registrars, general practitioners, psychologists, nurses and physiotherapists. It is written by two hospital consultants responsible for running Pain Clinics in general hospitals, with two chapters provided by a colleague in a neurosurgical centre.

What is chronic pain?

A definition that describes a chronic condition as a long-standing acute condition is inadequate. Tissues involved in chronic inflammation, for example, can be distinguished microscopically from those with acute inflammation by changes of regeneration and repair. Once a condition becomes chronic, secondary changes make for an immediate situation in which management involves treating complications of the condition rather than the condition itself. Thus it is with chronic pain. Chronic pain is not a symptom of an illness. It is an illness. It has its own symptoms, signs and complications. The professional caring for the chronic pain sufferer looks for complications of chronic pain and attempts to treat these. The original cause of the chronic pain may be irrelevant. If there is a possible cure the professional is advised to ascertain the degree to which the complications of chronic pain have become apparent: the complications themselves may seriously limit the benefit that might otherwise be obtained from treatment of the pain.

This book

The opening chapters explain the terms with which the professional should be familiar, and some of the practical problems encountered in Pain Clinic practice. They should be read as an introduction. Elsewhere the book is arranged according to topics in alphabetical order, in the format familiar to readers of the series. Cross-reference may be made to other chapters. The chapters on cancer pain are kept together.

We have attempted to organize our topics so that evidence-based medicine is afforded high priority. Yet we accept that much of our practice, and that of those with whom we meet regularly to share clinical problems, is based on precedent and experience. Our sources include comments made by colleagues in lectures at national and international meetings, and informally. It is impossible to acknowledge all of these sources.

The book is dedicated to our trainees and those other professionals who have laboured with us to build up our respective practices. In particular we acknowledge the support of Chris Glynn, Sara Severn, Frank Grady, Alan Severn and Barrie Tait.

Names of Medical Substances

In accordance with directive 92/27/EEC, this book adheres to the following guidelines on naming of medicinal substances (rINN, Recommended International Non-proprietary Name; BAN, British Approved Name).

List 1 – Both names to appear

UK Name	rINN
[1]adrenaline	epinephrine
amethocaine	tetracaine
bendrofluazide	bendroflumethiazide
benzhexol	trihexyphenidyl
chlorpheniramine	chlorphenamine
dicyclomine	dicycloverine
dothiepin	dosulepin
eformoterol	formoterol
flurandrenolone	fludroxycortide
frusemide	furosemide
hydroxyurea	hydroxycarbamide
lignocaine	lidocaine
methotrimeprazine	levomepromazine
methylene blue	methylthioninium chloride
mitozantrone	mitoxantrone
mustine	chlormethine
nicoumalone	acenocoumarol
[1]noradrenaline	norepinephrine
oxypentifylline	pentoxyifylline
procaine penicillin	procaine benzylpenicillin
salcatonin	calcitonin (salmon)
thymoxamine	moxisylyte
thyroxine sodium	levothyroxine sodium
trimeprazine	alimemazine

List 2 – rINN to appear exclusively

Former BAN	rINN/new BAN
amoxycillin	amoxicillin
amphetamine	amfetamine
amylobarbitone	amobarbital
amylobarbitone sodium	amobarbital sodium
beclomethasone	beclometasone
benorylate	benorilate
busulphan	busulfan
butobarbitone	butobarbital
carticaine	articane
cephalexin	cefalexin
cephamandole nafate	cefamandole nafate
cephazolin	cefazolin
cephradine	cefradine
chloral betaine	cloral betaine
chlorbutol	chlorobutanol
chlormethiazole	clomethiazole
chlorathalidone	chlortalidone
cholecalciferol	colecalciferol
cholestyramine	colestyramine
clomiphene	clomifene
colistin sulphomethate sodium	colistimethate sodium
corticotrophin	corticotropin
cysteamine	mercaptamine
danthron	dantron
desoxymethasone	desoximetasone
dexamphetamine	dexamfetamine
dibromopropamidine	dibrompropamidine
dienoestrol	dienestrol
dimethicone(s)	dimeticone
dimethyl sulphoxide	dimethyl sulfoxide
doxycycline hydrochloride (hemihydrate hemiethanolate)	doxycycline hyclate
ethancrynic acid	etacrynic acid
ethamsylate	etamsylate
ethinyloestradiol	ethinylestradiol
ethynodiol	etynodiol
flumethasone	flumetasone
flupenthixol	flupentixol
gestronol	gestonorone
guaiphenesin	guaifenesin
hexachlorophane	hexachlorophene

[1]In common with the BP, precedence will continue to be given to the terms adrenaline and noradrenaline.

hexamine hippurate	methenamine hippurate	riboflavine	riboflavin
hydroxyprogesterone hexanoate	hydroxyprogesterone caproate	sodium calciumedetate	sodium calcium edetate
		sodium cromoglycate	sodium cromoglicate
indomethacin	indometacin	sodium ironedetate	sodium feredetate
lysuride	lisuride	sodium picosulphate	sodium picosulfate
methyl cysteine	mecysteine	sorbitan monostearate	sorbitan stearate
methylphenobarbitone	methylphenobarbital	stilboestrol	diethylstilbestrol
oestradiol	estradiol	sulphacetamide	sulfacetamide
oestriol	estriol	sulphadiazine	sulfadiazine
oestrone	estrone	sulphadimidine	sulfadimidine
oxethazaine	oxetacaine	sulphaguanadine	sulfaguanadine
pentaerythritol tetranitrate	pentaerithrityl tetranitrate	sulphamethoxazole	sulfamethoxazole
		sulphasalazine	sulfasalazine
phenobarbitone	phenobarbital	sulphathiazole	sulfathiazole
pipothiazine	pipotiazine	sulphinpyrazone	sulfinpyrazone
polyhexanide	polihexanide	tetracosactrin	tetracosactide
potassium cloazepate	dipotassium clorazepate	thiabendazole	tiabendazole
pramoxine	pramocaine	thioguanine	tioguanine
prothionamide	protionamide	thiopentone	thiopental
quinalbarbitone	secobarbital	urofollitrophin	urofollitropin

DEDICATION

To the memory of Daniel and with thanks to all those who supported his family. Effective pain and symptom relief enabled him to lead a full and active life.

INTRODUCTION – WHAT ARE PAIN SERVICES?

Scope of pain medicine and the professions involved

Chronic pain patients are a diverse group of patients. Historically, the major impetus for the establishment of specialist pain clinics was cancer pain and the development of techniques for nerve destruction, using techniques refined from specialist local anaesthetic practice. However, improvement in medical management and nursing care of cancer patients has in most cases superseded the need for techniques that prompted such specialist interest. The focus of attention of many pain clinics has thus become one of managing a condition that is usefully called a chronic pain syndrome, rather than the treatment of pain symptoms. The general hospital pain clinic manages cancer pain, nerve injury pain, chronic back problems and peripheral vascular disease. Its involvement may be for technical service reasons, such as a sympathectomy to improve blood flow to the ischaemic limb, or it may take the lead role in managing the complex medical and psychosocial problem called the chronic pain syndrome.

Acute pain services may exist together with the chronic pain service or be separate in terms of personnel and management, and be responsible for the development of policies for pain management on surgical and medical wards as well as the education of staff and the direct clinical care of specific patients. In the United Kingdom the Royal College of Anaesthetists has established a Faculty of Pain Medicine responsible for the training of medically qualified anaesthesia specialists. The British Pain Society is the UK chapter of the International Association for the Study of Pain (IASP), an organization which has members from many professions, many of whom have their own postgraduate training schemes.

Pain as a disease

The chronic pain syndrome is the end result of a variety of pathological and psychological mechanisms that may have included, at some stage, tissue or nerve damage, and in which symptoms have failed to resolve with healing or repair. It is helpful to consider the chronic pain syndrome as a disease in its own right. Chronic pain syndrome has its own symptomatology, signs and natural history that can be recognized in many patients irrespective of the primary source of the symptoms of pain. The management of the chronic pain syndrome requires the clinician to shift emphasis from the relief of the pain to the prevention of complications and the rehabilitation of the sufferer, a role similar to that of a physician managing any other chronic condition. Symptomatic relief is of less importance than the development of a strategy for long-term management. While it is noted that short-term relief of pain symptoms is reported with many techniques, both 'conventional' and 'complementary', the prospects of these interventions to deliver long-lasting changes in function and behaviour are by no means as certain. Indeed, there are risks of any technique that provides short-term relief but does not address the consequences of chronic pain, namely that the sufferer relies on the professional for repeated intervention. In practice this means that establishment of a service providing a low-cost, minimally invasive modality of treatment, for example, using acupuncture, commits the clinician to a long-term, open-ended relationship with the patient unless some form of 'contract' is agreed with the patient. Agreement has to be made with patient and health care purchaser that sees a course of treatment designed not only to provide symptomatic relief but also to reduce disability and encourage a return to normal activity. One way of assessing the effectiveness of treatment is to shift the line of enquiry from 'did it hurt less?' to 'did you manage to do more?'. It is important that the patient understands this role. The patient needs to be aware of his or her own responsibility to maintain any gains which have been achieved in the pain clinic.

The contract between pain clinic and the purchaser of the service must therefore reflect the type and extent of rehabilitation work that needs to be undertaken by the pain clinic. Features that have to be addressed are the length of time for which follow up is necessary and the number and role of other professions that need to be formally involved. The growth in number and variety of interested professionals means that there is no one model of care provision that needs to be accepted as 'standard'. Without standardization it is difficult to decide on an outcome that allows the patient to be returned from the supervision of the clinic to the supervision of the primary care team. Desired outcomes will vary, depending on the type of referral and the ability of primary care to take on responsibility for long-term monitoring. It is to be expected that there will be frequent requests for review of the pain symptoms and advice on management of the condition of chronic pain.

Relationship with other medical bodies

Investigation of ongoing pathology is not the role of the clinic, although a working knowledge of screening for and referral of suspected rheumatological and neurological disease is required. This is best obtained by discussion with local specialists. Similarly, local negotiation will define the limits of responsibility for the management of conditions such as headache, back pain, osteoporosis and cancer. In general terms, attendance at the chronic pain clinic assumes that all reasonable attempts at diagnosis and management of ongoing disease have been addressed by relevant specialists. Some acceptance of the unique role of the clinic as a resource for the management of a chronic condition is however desirable. It may be convenient for a pain clinic to take on the major role for symptom relief from other specialists, for example for the performing of procedures such as epidural injections, but the wider need for rehabilitation in this group of patients must not be lost in the press of referrals for interventions with only short-term proven benefit.

Clinical governance

Clinical governance is a doctrine that the clinician is responsible to the employing authority, as well as his professional body, for aspects of professional conduct. The pain clinician may therefore expect to be involved in advising the employer about issues concerning the management of patients under the care of colleagues, and in advising about policies that may affect many patients. Conversely, it is important that where clinical experience dictates the use of an approach or techniques for which high-level evidence is unavailable or unconvincing, appropriate measures are taken to ensure that clinical and management colleagues are aware of the clinical reasoning. Prescribing outside a manufacturer's product licence is a case in point. In this case it may be valuable that the employer endorses the practice after consideration by a Drugs and Therapeutics Committee or similar. The consultant has a special responsibility for monitoring the patient on unlicensed medication that may be difficult to delegate to primary care, a trainee, or a nurse.

Pain clinics treat patients who may have failed to respond to conventional medical treatments carried out by other specialists. Some of them have complaints about the way in which they have been treated, others about the complications of which they believe that they were not warned. Although the complaint itself may require investigation and an appropriate answer, the process of complaining may be part of the presentation of the disease. The employer therefore has to be prepared to recognize that over-solicitous apology for an alleged inaction may reinforce the behaviour and lead to repeated frustrations and complaints.

Relationship with non-medical bodies

The clinician is encouraged to extend influence beyond the immediate medical community to the self-help groups that meet outside hospitals. Many of them understand the strategy of management of chronic pain. Some do not, and may have as their *raison d'être* a commitment to see the provision of a service which is at odds with the clinician's professional judgement. The influence of such groups may be considerable, particularly when they are well organized, skilfully administered, registered as charities, and have the support of well-known personalities. These groups have more information available to them through the Internet, and may have access through this medium to 'specialists' whose views may be very different from the local clinic. The clinician is advised not to ignore the local impact and support that these groups often have, even if some conflict is involved. It is well worth finding out what groups exist, what access there is to information on the Internet and where the agenda of the group differs from that of the clinician. Common grounds for mutual support may be found, even when there is disagreement about some aspects of the aims of the group. Similarly, such groups may be considered allies in the quest for resources, although the clinician must keep the aims of the group subject to his/her professional judgement when deciding what types of treatment should be provided with such resources.

Medicolegal reporting

The role of the legal system is to decide what is genuine and to compensate appropriately where there is blame. The area of chronic pain presents problems in trying to do this. For those without understanding of pain and its mechanisms, the concept of pain following injury that does not resolve after tissue healing is difficult to grasp. Further difficulty arises because chronic pain is often reported where there is no obvious pathology. Moreover, chronic pain in itself manifests a variety of psychological features and behavioural adaptations or 'inconsistencies' which may be perceived as fraudulent or malingering behaviour. At the centre of the legal problem is the question: 'Is the patient attempting to deceive or exaggerate?' There is no way to know. However, although the report of pain may be said to be entirely subjective, for those with specialist knowledge there may be features in the history which give objectivity, as they are spontaneous reports of what the patient would be unlikely to know: e.g. 'it's numb but it hurts' or, on examination, the demonstration of allodynia. It remains, however, that there are pains for which there is no objective evidence and this group will always be questioned as genuine.

The very specialized duty of the pain clinician to the court in medicolegal reporting of chronic pain cases is to provide assessment of presence and degree of pain by the professional interpretation of history and signs on examination, to provide explanation as to why a pain may be ongoing and to describe the 'normal' features of a chronic pain syndrome. Illness behaviour can be thought of as an expression that the patient is suffering pain.

ANATOMY AND PHYSIOLOGY

The sensory system for pain consists of a population of receptors, primary afferent neurones, neurones of the dorsal root of the spinal cord and a pathway to the midbrain, thalamus and cortex via the spinothalamic tract on the opposite side of the spinal cord. Knowledge of the anatomy of pain pathways (a result of studies of cases with damage to nerve pathways and experimental observation) is detailed, but understanding of how the behaviour of the sensory system for pain changes with nerve damage or persistent stimulation is rudimentary. In contrast to the other sensory systems, pain is not a line-labelled, modality-specific, hard-wired system, but one in which the relationship between input (stimulus) and output (response) is variable. This variability has led to the development of 'models', to explain the sensory system for pain. Models are theoretical systems that describe the workings of the central nervous system in a simple way that matches certain, but not all, observed clinical and neurophysiological phenomena. An example of such a model is the gate control model, described by Melzack and Wall in 1967. No models are comprehensive representations of the complex processing systems of the sensory system for pain, but they are useful provided that their limitations are understood. The gate control model, for example, explains how physical activities such as rubbing the skin can alleviate the pain of arthritis or a nettle sting, but it does not explain why patients with postherpetic neuralgia may be unable to tolerate the same activity.

Anatomy and physiology

Nociceptors

Receptors which respond to painful stimuli are termed nociceptors. They are simple nerve endings devoid of the elaborate organization found in the sensory systems for pressure and position sense. They respond to strong thermal and mechanical stimuli. Despite their similar ultrastructural appearance, they are not a homogeneous population, and their ability to propagate nerve impulses changes with their environment.

Silent nociceptors

Silent nociceptors are nociceptors which are inactive in the resting state and apparently refractory to mechanical or electrical stimuli. However, in the presence of tissue damage or chemical mediators of inflammation these nociceptors become active. It is believed that, although 'silent' from the perspective of nerve impulse propagation, these nociceptors provide the sensory system with continuous data about the tissue environment. This information is signalled to the spinal cord via microtubular transport mechanisms in the axon.

Primary afferent fibres

Primary afferent fibres are described as A or C fibres on the basis of microscopic appearance and velocity of conduction of electrical impulses. A fibres are larger, are well insulated by myelin and conduct impulses at high velocity. C fibres are smaller, poorly insulated and conduct impulses slowly. The population of A fibres seen in a microscopic preparation of a nerve is subdivided by size into:

- Aα – motor nerves.
- Aβ – sensory nerves for light touch and vibration.
- Aγ – motor nerves.
- Aδ – sensory nerves for pain.

A and C fibres have different actions at the dorsal horn of the spinal cord.

'Models' of sensory processing in nociception

Descartes model (17th Century)

Descartes recognized the role of the spinal cord in communicating information from the site of injury to the brain. The spinal cord was believed to consist of a series of hollow tubes which had an intrinsic property of being able to modulate the intensity of the signals they passed to the brain.

Specificity model

Histological studies of skin and joint capsules demonstrate the presence of specialized nerve endings responsible for diverse sensory functions such as pressure and joint position sense. The specificity model proposed that pain was signalled by specialist nerve endings along well-defined nerve pathways.

Summation model

The antithesis of the specificity model, the summation model proposed that nociception was the result of a barrage of stimulation of all modalities of sensory fibres, and that, for example, excess stimulation of a specific receptor (for example, one which responds to pressure) would be experienced as pain. Experimentally it can be shown that a painful sensation is experienced if mild heat and cold stimuli are delivered by specialist quantitative sensory testing equipment to adjacent areas of skin.

Gate control model

This model described the relationship between nociceptive and tactile afferents in the dorsal horn as an electronic switch in order to explain variability between input and output in the sensory system for pain. The model was also used to explain the influence of higher centres of control on the experience of pain, based on observations in 1944 by the military surgeon Beecher on the battlefield at Anzio, Italy. According to this model, Aβ afferents and descending inhibitory pathways inhibit dorsal horn neurones from responding to Aδ- and C-fibre inputs. The gate control model reconciles some of the contradictions between the earlier models in that it recognizes the signalling characteristics of a specific group of neurones that can be modified by interactions with other neurones. It is also worth noting that Descartes had earlier recognized the observation for which Melzack, Wall and Beecher take credit: that the nervous system has an ability to regulate the intensity of the pain experience.

Neuronal sensitization model

This model described the result of changes in the environment of nociceptor or dorsal horn spinal cord cell to tissue damage or persistent stimulation. It is described as 'peripheral' where it affects the primary afferent neurone and 'central' where it affects the dorsal horn.

1. Peripheral sensitization results from a change in the local receptor environment. There are several possible mediators of the process of sensitization, and they are present in areas of inflammation. They may act alone or in combination, and by direct action on the nerve ending or by a process of sensitizing the nociceptor to mechanical and thermal stimuli.

The mediators include:

- H^+ ions.
- K^+ ions.
- Bradykinin.
- Serotonin.
- Prostaglandins.
- Neurokinins.

A consequence of the process of sensitization is that myelinated Aβ fibres, those which form part of the gate control model, change their activity, and by a mechanism which is poorly understood, cease to function as inhibitors of dorsal horn activity.

2. Central sensitization describes the changes in the dorsal horn neurone when it is stimulated by the primary afferent neurone, either by a low-grade continuous C-fibre stimulation of a nociceptive process, or following the increased activity from damaged nerves in neuropathic pain. A-fibre discharges cause transient changes at the synapse between primary afferent and spinal cord neurones. C-fibre discharges cause prolonged, progressive and ultimately irreversible changes.

The increased excitability of the dorsal horn neurone that results from chronic repetitive C-fibre stimulation has been studied in isolated spinal cord preparations where it is termed 'windup'. Central sensitization is the clinical manifestation of this increased physiological activity.

Neuromatrix model

Any model which tries to explain brain mechanisms in chronic pain must consider the diverse and detailed sensations of which a patient with a complete transection of the spinal cord lesion can complain. Such descriptions support the theory of a central pain-generating area, part of a 'neuromatrix' within the brain responsible for both the sensation and its associated emotional and psychological sequelae, but triggered by nociceptive stimuli or inappropriate neuropathic stimuli. Thus, a patient with a spinal cord transection may not only be aware of a phantom sensation such as bicycling but may also suffer phantom muscle cramps and fatigue with time if the sensation persists. The idea of the brain having an intrinsic ability to create its own experience of pain is helpful for patients and clinicians to understand failure when therapy targeted at peripheral causes has failed. The neuromatrix model differs from earlier models which gave an anatomical basis to the nerve pathways from the periphery. The neuromatrix model is supported by the new imaging technologies of functional magnetic resonance imaging (fMRI), and positron emission tomography (PET). Both are safe, non-invasive techniques.

fMRI. Functional MRI detects the **b**lood **o**xygen **l**evel-**d**ependent (BOLD) changes in the MRI signal that arise when changes in neuronal activity occur following a stimulus or task. An increase in neural activity in a region of cortex stimulates an increase in the local blood flow. The supply actually exceeds the demand, so that at the capillary level there is a net increase in the proportion of oxygenated arterial blood to deoxygenated venous blood and the concentration of deoxyhaemoglobin within the tissue falls. This decrease has a direct effect on the signals, since deoxyhaemoglobin is significantly paramagnetic. The result of having lower levels of deoxyhaemoglobin in blood in a region of brain tissue is that the MRI signal from that region decays less rapidly and so is stronger when it is recorded in a typical magnetic resonance image acquisition. This small signal increase is the BOLD signal recorded in fMRI, with the 'active' areas of the cortex 'lightening' up.

PET detects areas of metabolism within the brain. A positron emitting tracer compound is synthesized and introduced into the bloodstream. The tracer may be any biologically relevant chemical – the most common one in use is FDG (fluorodeoxyglucose), which is a marker of metabolism. It distributes according to metabolism. Thus, in the brain, in a pain state, it will localize specifically to an area of brain active in pain processing. In the decay process, two positrons are emitted in opposite directions; thus, in a detector the location of such an event is indicated by a coincident positron, one arriving at two detectors 180° apart simultaneously. By this means the various parts of the pain matrix have been identified: the lateral component deals with the location, severity and modality of the sensory stimulus, and the medial component of the matrix deals more with the affective, emotional, memory and cognitive components of the pain experience.

Until the advent of non-invasive human brain imaging, our understanding of the role of the brain in pain processing was limited. We do know that the perception of pain due to an injury or in clinical pain states undergoes substantial processing at supraspinal levels and, increasingly, these supraspinal mechanisms are recognized as playing a major role in the representation and modulation of the pain experience. Functional neuroimaging of the pain experience provides a unique instrument for better understanding of pain. We can now assert the role of the cortex in pain perception and, instead of localizing a singular 'pain centre' in the brain, neuroimaging studies identify a matrix of somatosensory (S1, S2, insular cortex), limbic (insular cortex, anterior cingulated cortex) and associated (prefrontal cortex) structures receiving parallel inputs from multiple nociceptive pathways.

The future role of fMRI will be the investigation of cortical representation of specific pain types, effect of therapy options and the possibility of modulating these regions via pharmacological and behavioural methods. One of the more intriguing aspects of this research is the use of fMRI to observe changes after psychological therapy. PET, likewise, has great potential – the possibility exists of labelling drugs to determine their sites of action or investigating receptor-binding properties.

Biopsychosocial model

The biopsychosocial model is an alternative way of looking at the experience of pain. Rather than seeing the pain as a symptom of a physical disorder, the model described a disease, the pain syndrome, as an entity in itself. The symptoms of the syndrome are such features as depressed mood, misunderstanding of the cause of the pain or its significance and unrealistic expectations of treatment. The signs of the condition are the behaviours associated with the symptoms, such as social withdrawal and avoidance of activity. The biopsychosocial model, like all others, explains some features of the experience of pain but not all. It has to be emphasized that the use of this model does not imply that the patient has a primary psychological illness.

Nociceptive and neuropathic pain: clinical correlates with mechanisms

The clinical distinction between nociceptive (tissue damage) pain and neuropathic (nerve damage) pain is valuable as it may help the clinician choose the appropriate therapy, and it is valuable for an understanding of the very complicated patterns of pain that can cause distress if not properly understood. The patient who complains of pain while being bewildered by cutaneous numbness or the loss of a limb may be reassured by understanding that neuropathic pain is a real phenomenon. However, rigid distinctions of pain as 'neuropathic' or 'nociceptive' may be as unhelpful as a rigid adherence to any one of the 'models' described above. Postherpetic neuralgia, for example, classically described as a neuropathic pain, in fact presents in some patients with an unpleasant mixture of neuropathic and nociceptive elements which may have to be separately accounted for in examination and assessment of the response to treatment. The recent demonstration that gabapentin can reduce postoperative opioid requirements may be another example of the distinction between nociceptive and neuropathic pain being blurred.

Thinking of the 'final common pathways' in pain processing, it is not difficult to understand why the two models of origin of pain are indistinct in certain cases. Minor trauma, such as a skin incision, causes damage to sensory nerve endings. Major trauma, such as an amputation, causes trauma to nerve trunks. Nerves have their own supply of nociceptors, the *nervi nervorum*, so nerve damage will be relayed to the spinal cord as a nociceptive signal. The output from the spinal cord to the brain will be influenced by central sensitization irrespective of the original source of the signal.

The sensitized state, which as we see above can exist in neuropathic conditions or in certain conditions where there is unrelieved nociceptive stimulation, has the following clinical features:

Spontaneous pain, which may be:

- Paroxysmal, with a quality described as burning, shooting or numb.
- Severe pain in response to a noxious stimulus (hyperalgesia).
- Severe pain in response to a stimulus which is not normally noxious (allodynia).
- Severe pain in response to stimulation despite sensory impairment (hyperpathia).

Where this occurs after nociceptive stimulation, hyperalgesia results from a change in the receptive properties of the nociceptor to tissue injury. Secondary hyperalgesia is a consequence of the temporal and spatial summation of nociceptor input into the spinal cord. Allodynia results from a change in the signalling characteristics of the Aβ fibres.

Neuropathic pain is associated with the following conditions:

- Surgical scar pain.
- Diabetic neuropathy.
- Complex regional pain syndromes.
- Postherpetic neuralgia.
- Polyneuropathies and neuralgia.
- Demyelination.
- Radicular pain associated with prolapsed intervertebral disc.
- Spinal cord injury.
- Stroke.

A damaged primary afferent fibre demonstrates three electrophysiological features which may contribute to the process of central sensitization and offer rationale for therapy:

- Spontaneous activity.
- Exaggerated response to stimulus.
- Sensitivity to catecholamines.

Spontaneous activity can develop at the site of damage, at a site of demyelination, or within the cell body of the damaged neurone in the dorsal root ganglion. Where damage to a neurone is incomplete, the primary afferent terminal itself may become spontaneously active. Spontaneous activity is influenced by the local environment: inflammatory mediators and noradrenaline increase the level of activity. As well as the changes that can be observed in damaged nerves, other disturbances of function are noted. An inflammatory response occurs. Undamaged nerve fibres are themselves sensitized by changes in adjacent damaged fibres: some of the more painful neuropathies are partial nerve lesions.

Sensitization: molecular mechanisms in nociceptive and neuropathic pain

Experimentally, the observation of C-fibre sensization of the dorsal horn neurone is described by the graphic term 'windup', implying an amplification of the output of the dorsal horn in response to constant low-intensity input from nociceptive afferents. Windup refers to the specific action of C fibres (that is nociceptive input) on the dorsal horn neurone. It is not known whether windup is a normal protective response or a pathological one. What is clear, however, is that under certain circumstances, unremitting nociceptive stimulation of the spinal cord leads to irreversible changes in the synaptic and cellular organization of the dorsal horn that persist after withdrawal of the stimulus.

C fibres release peptides (substance P and neurokinin A) and amino acids (glutamate and aspartate) on to dorsal horn neurones. Dorsal horn neurones have receptors for neurokinin and glutamate, the latter being the N-methyl-D-aspartic acid (NMDA) receptor, which in the resting state is refractory to stimulation. Its transition to a state in which it responds to glutamate is accomplished by the interaction of substance P with the neurokinin receptor. Subsequent C-fibre stimulation leads to glutamate-mediated NMDA activation and an enhanced response to the afferent stimulus. The dorsal horn neurone is said to be sensitized. In its sensitized state secondary changes in other neurotransmitter receptor systems and membrane proteins occur. Interest has been expressed in the voltage-sensitive calcium channels (VSCCs). In the resting state these ion channels are sensitive to morphine, whose action is to reduce the flow of calcium through the channel. However, this morphine sensitivity of the VSCC is lost in the sensitized dorsal horn neurone. Similarly, there are changes in the process of signalling between large-fibre light-touch neurones and the dorsal horn after sensitization. It is said that the changes in the nervous system with sensitization are analogous to those of early fetal development; in other words, sensitization involves a regression of neuronal signalling to a more 'primitive' type. Biochemical and protein synthesis changes after sensitization can be observed by measuring the appearance of products of the expression of the *c-fos* gene. This indicates synthesis of nerve growth factor and neurotransmitters within the sensitized neurone. There are other biochemical changes, most notably reduction of substance P and calcitonin gene-related peptide (CGRP) synthesis, and increased neuropeptide Y and vasoactive intestinal peptide synthesis.

It is of note that the analgesic drug ketamine is an antagonist of the NMDA receptor, although it is not known, for reasons discussed above, whether such a drug has a role in the prophylaxis of neuropathic pain. Similarly, the concept of preemptive analgesia in acute pain management bases its reasoning on the thesis that inhibition of nociceptor input (and neuropathic input in the case of amputation pain) prior to trauma, will prevent sensitization.

Further reading

Fields HL, Rowbotham MC. Multiple mechanisms of neuropathic pain: a clinical perspective. In: Gebhart GF, Hammond DL, Jensen TS (eds). Proceedings of the 7th World Congress on Pain, Paris. Seattle: IASP Press, 1994; pp. 437–54.

Melzack R. Central pain syndromes and theories of pain. In: Casey KL (ed.). Pain and Central Nervous System Disease: The Central Pain Syndromes. New York: Raven Press, 1991; 59–64.

APPLYING EVIDENCE IN CLINICAL PRACTICE

Evidence-based medicine

The ideas of evidence-based medicine (EBM) arose from the writings of the Scottish epidemiologist Archie Cochrane, most famously his book *Effectiveness and Efficiency*, first published in 1972. These were taken up and publicized by David Sackett and colleagues at McMaster University in Canada in the late 1970s and 1980s. Cochrane argued that much of medical practice was not based on good scientific evidence, and suggested that the randomized controlled trial (RCT) be used more widely to show which interventions were beneficial and which were not.

There are five simple steps to practising EBM:

1. *Ask a clinical question you can answer.* A good question specifies intervention, comparison, subjects and outcome.
2. *Search for evidence.* Usually on computerized databases such as Medline.
3. *Critically appraise the evidence.* Is the research of good quality? Are the results important and useful for me as a clinician?
4. *Integrate the evidence into practice.* Decide how (or if) it applies to the patient.
5. *Evaluate the process.* Did it work? Could we have done it better?

Now the idea of going back to primary sources of research to answer clinical questions is not new. What is novel, however, is the exhortation that ordinary doctors and other health care workers should do it for themselves rather than rely on others. This brings with it great potential benefits.

Evidence-based medicine offers at once a way of making the medical literature more manageable, a way of answering problems arising in clinical practice, a way of keeping up to date and a way of finding what helps patients and what does not. However, it needs skills for each step that many clinicians do not have or feel diffident about using. There is ample guidance on how to develop such skills (see Further Reading) and here I offer some general suggestions.

Evidence can be sought from primary sources, i.e. by finding the original research papers. However, the process of implementing evidence-based practice can be made easier by using sources of pre-appraised evidence that present summaries of critically appraised evidence, systematic reviews and other collations of information. Some useful general sources include:

- ACP Journal Club (www.acpjc.org).
- Clinical Evidence (www.clinicalevidence.com).
- Bandolier (www.jr2.ox.ac.uk/bandolier).
- The Cochrane Library (www.thecochranelibrary.com).
- UK National Institute for Clinical Excellence (NICE) (www.nice.org.uk).

Readers need to be aware, however, whether such publications represent pure 'evidence' or, in the case of some NICE guidance, the evidence 'interpreted' by consensus groups. Although this is quite acceptable, it should always be made clear.

The *Cochrane Library* is worthy of particular mention. In 1979, Archie Cochrane challenged the medical profession to put together, by specialty, a critical summary of RCTs to enable medical practice to be put on a sounder footing of evidence. The Cochrane Collaboration evolved from this and is now a world-wide venture whose aims are to prepare, maintain and disseminate systematic reviews of the effects of health care interventions. As well as thousands of completed systematic reviews and protocols, the Cochrane Library also contains the Database of Abstracts of Reviews of Effectiveness (high-quality reviews from non-Cochrane sources), and the Controlled Clinical Trials Register, with over 470 000 clinical trials. The Cochrane Library is updated every 3 months on CD-ROM and is also available on line. Further information can be found at www.cochrane.org. In the United Kingdom, staff within the NHS should be able to access the full text of reviews through the National Library for Health. Most areas of health care are now represented, and reviews dealing with chronic pain have found their way into the Cochrane Library through various review groups – for instance, the Musculoskeletal Group maintains the reviews on interventions for low back pain. There is, however, a Cochrane Pain, Palliative and Supportive Care Group, which had 54 completed reviews and 43 protocols published in November 2005. An up-to-date list of reviews, protocols and registered titles can be found at www.cochrane.no/titles or through the Group's website below.

The group is based in Oxford, and correspondence should be addressed to:

Jessica Thomas
Review Group Co-ordinator
Pain Research Unit
Churchill Hospital
Oxford OX3 7LJ
UK

E-mail: jessica.thomas@pru.ox.ac.uk

www.jr2.ox.ac.uk/cochrane

Making sense of the evidence

Levels of evidence

The idea of a hierarchy of evidence is now quite well known. A typical, simple example is shown as Table 1. If you have to make a treatment decision, you should choose a therapy whose effectiveness has been demonstrated by a well-conducted systematic review. Failing that, it should be supported by a sound RCT. Beyond that, the evidence from the different types of study is thought to be less and less robust – that is, potentially more biased and less reliable – as you move down the order.

Table 1. Typical hierarchy of evidence

I	Systematic review of RCT
II	Single RCT
III	Observational studies, e.g. cohort studies
IV	Case series
V	Case report

Although it remains true that the RCT – and hence, quantitative meta-analyses derived from an RCT – provide the best available current evidence for effectiveness of therapies, they are not the best way of answering every question arising from our clinical practice. For instance, many RCTs do not examine adverse effects of treatments, and these can be important in determining patient compliance. Conversely, case reports do not provide a powerful basis for the effectiveness of a treatment but can be very useful for publicizing complications such as adverse drug reactions.

The randomized controlled trial

The RCT has been used in medicine since the 1940s. Improvements in methodology mean that, for appropriate research questions, results can be obtained with a very low risk of bias.

As time has passed, the methodological rigour of clinical investigations has increased. Whereas uncontrolled observational studies of new treatments were once the norm, random allocation into one or more groups is now standard practice. Some element of blinding, i.e. hiding from patients, their doctors and sometimes others, which group patients are in, is usual. These two steps – allocation concealment and blinding – are thought to be the two most important ways of reducing bias. Non-randomized studies tend to overestimate the effects of new treatments when compared with placebo.

The systematic review

Essentially, a systematic review is a pre-planned investigation in itself. If one were planning a clinical trial, one would set out in advance, in the form of a protocol, what the research question was, who would be studied, how the results would be analysed and so on. The systematic review uses the same principles. The term *secondary research* is often used to describe the science of systematic reviews, to contrast it with the primary studies on which the reviews are based. This is useful because it connotes a more methodical approach, but also because it implies by association that biases can creep in here, just as they can into an RCT. Particular biases that need to be avoided include:

- Publication bias (journals are more likely to publish studies with positive than negative results).
- Language bias (many reviewers search only for English language material).
- Appraisal bias (subjective criteria used for judging study quality).
- Inference bias (the conclusions are not supported by the results!).

Perhaps the biggest benefit of the systematic approach is that it makes the review process more transparent and allows readers to see how the conclusions were reached and hence judge for themselves how useful they are.

Making sense of numerical expressions of the results of research

This first example uses a fictitious RCT of a new anticonvulsant, gabatryptiline, for the treatment of neuropathic pain. In all, 1092 patients took part, of whom 529 received the active treatment and 563 the control drug. The outcome in question is a 50% reduction in severity of pain. Of the patients taking gabatryptiline, 378 responded, as opposed to 303 of those taking the control drug. Table 2 expresses these results in a 2 × 2 table.

Table 2. RCT of a new anticonvlsant

	Responded	Did not respond	Total
Active	378	151	529
Control	303	260	563
Total	681	411	1092

The **risk** (or probability) of having pain in the gabatryptiline group is 151/529, which is 0.29.

The **baseline risk** of having pain (control group) is 260/563, which is 0.46.

The **risk ratio** (or **relative risk**) is the gabatryptiline risk divided by the baseline risk, i.e. 0.29/0.46, which works out at 0.63. This can also be expressed as relative benefit, which will be the reciprocal of the relative risk.

The **odds** of having pain in the gabatryptiline group are 151/378, which is 0.4.

The **baseline odds** of having pain are 260/303, which is 0.86.

The **odds ratio** is the gabatryptiline odds divided by the baseline odds, i.e. 0.4/0.86, which works out at 0.46.

If the outcome in question is rare, the risk ratio and the odds ratio are numerically similar. As the observed outcome becomes more frequent (as it is in this example), their values diverge.

The **absolute risk reduction** is calculated by subtracting the gabatryptiline risk from the baseline risk, that is 0.46 – 0.29, which is 0.17 or 17%.

The **relative risk reduction** is calculated by subtracting the gabatryptiline risk from the baseline risk and dividing by the baseline risk, i.e. (0.46 – 0.29)/0.46. This works out at 0.37 or 37%.

The **number needed to treat** (NNT) tells us how many patients need to be treated with gabatryptiline for one to benefit. It is simply the reciprocal of the absolute risk reduction, or 1/0.17, which works out at 6.

An analagous measure is the **number needed to harm** (NNH). Although, in this example, as often happens in clinical trials of new agents, no attempt has been made to quantify adverse effects, this gives a measure of how commonly patients experience side effects. For instance, an NNH of 5 for drowsiness means that, on average, 1 patient will feel drowsy for every 5 patients taking the drug.

So the same results from the same trial can be expressed in a number of different ways. It has been shown that doctors, patients and policymakers do not always understand the significance of these different formats. The relative risk reduction of 37%, for instance, sounds much more impressive, and is likely to sell more gabatryptiline, than an absolute risk reduction of 17%, but they mean the same. However, they both convey more than the odds ratio to the uninitiated reader.

The number needed to treat, on the other hand, has become popular – and is widely used in this book – because it combines an easily-understood concept with the level-headed sobriety of the absolute risk reduction. It is useful in answering the question '*how well* does a treatment work?' rather than simply whether it works or not. It usefully encapsulates the therapeutic effort needed to get a therapeutic result. Numbers needed to treat for treatment (as opposed to prophylaxis) should be small – we expect large effects in small numbers of people. Because few treatments are 100% effective, and because few controls – even placebo or no treatment – are without some effects, NNT for effective treatments are usually in the range of 2–4. The use of NNT also allows a comparison of different drugs, even though they may not have been compared directly in the same clinical study. For instance, numbers needed to treat have been calculated for a number of analgesics in acute pain and have allowed the construction of a 'league table'. For instance, paracetamol 1 g with codeine 60 mg is at the top of the table, with an NNT of 2 (to achieve 50% pain relief), whereas tramadol 75 mg, with a NNT of 5, cannot be recommended so strongly.

Table 3 is a 'real-life' example taken from the Oxford analgesic league tables (see 'Further Reading' below for the website address). It shows the numbers needed to treat and relative benefit (the obverse of the relative risk) for anticonvulsants compared with placebo for neuropathic pain conditions.

Table 3. Analysis of trials of anticonvulsants vs placebo for neuropathic pain conditions

Condition	Number of trials	Anticonvulsant improved/total	Placebo improved/ total	Relative benefit (95% CI)	NNT (95% CI)
Diabetic neuropathy	3	56/68	26/68	1.9 (1.4–2.7)	2.5 (1.8–4.0)
Trigeminal neuralgia	3	178/315	41/224	3.1 (2.3–4.1)	2.6 (2.2–3.3)
Migraine prophylaxis	2	63/74	17/77	3.7 (2.4–5.9)	1.6 (1.3–2.0)
Other pain syndromes	1	5/14	1/15	5.4 (0.7–40)	Not calculated

CI, confidence interval; NNT, numbers needed to treat.
Reproduced with permission of Bandolier
(www.jr2.ox.ac.uk/bandolier/booth/painpag/Acutrev/Analgesics/leagtab.html).

The 'headline' figures for relative benefit and NNT are of course aggregates derived from a number of patients who show varying responses to treatment. Often, statistical tests are used to examine whether the overall average difference between two groups is significant, and this is usually expressed as a 'p value'. This is falling out of favour, as it addresses the question 'Which treatment is better on average?' when what we often want to know is 'How might the treatment work in my patient?' This is where the confidence intervals (95% CI) give an idea of the likely range of possible responses to treatment, and for this and other reasons they are increasingly preferred in the numerical expression of the results of research.

Integrating evidence and practice

Having levels of evidence in our minds, as they are throughout this book, is all very well and good, but what if the patient presents with a condition for which there is no good evidence from systematic reviews or RCTs? So-called lower levels of evidence may then have to suffice, and if this constitutes the best available evidence then that is all we can hope for – until something better comes along in the future. But whatever the type of study, simply making numerical sense of it is not enough. The results may be valid but, for them to be useful in practice, we need to know how applicable they are to our own patients. This is usually referred to as *generalizability*, but in fact might be better termed *individualizability*. There should be a clear description in the 'Methods' section of the study what sort of patients were included, so that readers can judge if they are similar. However, each patient is different, and whether the results of the study should be used in a given individual goes beyond simple evidence and also incorporates clinicians' and patients' values and preferences.

Sometimes, however, there really is no evidence and we are thrown back on our clinical judgement and compassion. Even when evidence is present, patients do not always welcome it. For many, the accumulated experience of a seasoned clinician is enough. And, worse, what if no effective treatment is available – when there is 'nothing more we can do?'. Although Archie Cochrane's name is now firmly associated with evidence-based medicine, he knew only too well, as medical officer in a prisoner-of-war camp in World War II, the importance of common kindness and humanity, as this extract from his autobiography, in which he attends to a dying Russian soldier, shows:

> ... The ward was full, so I put him in my room as he was moribund and screaming and I did not want to wake the ward. I examined him. He had obvious gross bilateral cavitation and a severe pleural rub. I thought the latter was the cause of the pain and screaming. I had no morphia, just aspirin, which had no effect. I felt desperate. I knew very little Russian then and there was no one in the ward who did. I finally instinctively sat down on the bed and took him in my arms, and the screaming stopped almost at once. He died peacefully in my arms a few hours later. It was not the pleurisy that caused the screaming, but loneliness. It was a wonderful education about the care of the dying.
> (From Cochrane AL. *One Man's Medicine: The Autobiography of Archie Cochrane*. London: British Medical Journal Memoir Club, 1988; reproduced with permission.)

Further reading

Analgesic league tables can be viewed at:
  http://www.jr2.ox.ac.uk/bandolier/booth/painpag/Acutrev/Analgesics/Leagtab.html

Bogardus ST, Holmboe E, Jekel JF. Perils, pitfalls and possibilities in talking about medical risk. Journal of the American Medical Association 1999; 281: 1037–41.

Egger M, Davey Smith G, Altman D, eds. Systematic Reviews in Health Care, 2nd edn. London: British Medical Journal Books, 2001.

Greenhalgh T. How to Read a Paper, 2nd edn. London: British Medical Journal Books, 2000.

Jadad AR. Randomised Controlled Trials. London: British Medical Journal Books, 1998.

Petticrew M. Systematic reviews from astronomy to zoology: myths and misconceptions. British Medical Journal 2001; 322: 98–101.

Sackett DL, Richardson WS, Rosenberg WM, et al. Evidence-Based Medicine. How to Practise and Teach EBM. Edinburgh: Churchill Livingstone, 1997.

Sterne JAC, Davey Smith G. Sifting the evidence – what's wrong with significance tests? British Medical Journal 2001; 322: 226–31.

Vandenbroucke JP. Case reports in an evidence-based world. Journal of the Royal Society of Medicine 1999; 92: 159–63.

ASSESSMENT OF CHRONIC PAIN – HISTORY

It is helpful to consider chronic pain as a disease in which many factors – physical, patho-logical and psychosocial – contribute to the presentation. Thus the history itself is more than the history of the symptoms which provide diagnostic clues, the traditional model on which medical science is based. The clinician taking a history of chronic pain must be prepared to set aside preconceptions on which traditional medical diagnosis is taught. For example, standard teaching may suggest that pain that is experienced in a 'glove' or 'stock-ing' distribution is in some way 'fraudulent' because it does not fit with a preconceived anatomical knowledge of the sensory dermatomes. From the perspective of the pain clinic, symptoms of pain should be recorded as they are experienced, without prejudice to the clinician's view of the mechanisms involved. Contributing psychosocial factors need to be noted, with the understanding that they are likely to be present, and in a way that the patient is not blamed for the presentation. Most importantly, since the aim of manage-ment of chronic pain is a reduction in disability and return of function, the history must include factors such as the impact of the pain on normal functioning. To achieve this the context of history taking is wide: patients, self-rating questionnaires, pain diagrams and diaries and the perspective of relatives all offer further information. Discussion of the pain with the patient allows psychological signs to be manifest. Although a diagnosis is less sought after in the pain clinic than in other settings, pathology better managed in other clinics has to be excluded. Traditional medical teaching identifies so-called screening 'red flags' in presentation of illness that mandate the focused search for serious pathology such as cancer or inflammatory disease. Pain clinic history taking uses an analogous screening technique for elements in the psychosocial presentation. We will refer to them as 'yellow flags' to distinguish them from the 'red flags': they are not life-threatening symptoms, but their presence means that the psychosocial history has to be clearly focused. They are symptoms that may need addressing in their own right with psychological treatments.

The pain

1. **The site** of pain may indicate an underlying local cause, a referred origin, a dermatomal or peripheral nerve distribution or may bear no relationship to traditional neuroanatomical patterns. The site of pain should be recorded as it is reported, without interpretation by the doctor as to the possible diagnosis.

2. **The nature.** Duration, rapidity of onset, whether a pain is intermittent or constant, how it varies in severity with time and circumstance and its overall progression or deterioration determine its nature.

3. **The character of pain** will point to its somatic, visceral or neuropathic component. Descriptions of nociceptive and neuropathic pain can be difficult to distinguish because of significant overlap of symptoms. The description may use words such as 'torturing' or 'cruel', that indicate a level of distress which may need formal evaluation.

4. Alleviating and exacerbating factors offer information about aetiology. All factors which have a bearing on pain should be considered. Pain that is reported as being relieved by rest may in certain circumstances be considered as a 'yellow flag'; pain affected by heat suggests a sympathetic nervous system component.

5. The severity of pain can be recorded as a numerical categorical scale score. In its simplest form this can be descriptive – the patient is asked, verbally, to rate the pain on an arbitrary numerical scale. Visual analogue scales are more sophisticated scoring systems in which the patient marks the score between two points on paper or a simple proprietary model, such as a thermometer.

6. The impact of pain is assessment of disability and social and personal incapacity caused by pain. It attempts to identify all factors affected by pain. Assessment of impact can contribute to the psychosocial assessment where it reveals personal gain which may result from continuing pain.

Treatments for pain

Details of all past treatments and their outcomes build a picture of the pain and avoid further futile attempts with the same modalities. However, history should determine whether treatment was effectively prescribed and whether compliance was adequate before considering it a failure. Current treatments and their effects should be noted. Patients may have beliefs about treatments which usefully contribute to psychological assessment, such as their condition being incurable because no treatment has ever worked, an unshakeable belief in a particular treatment and unreasonable expectations from treatments they have not yet tried. These features are 'yellow flags'.

Other medical history

Other symptoms or conditions can have a bearing on the pain itself or on proposed pain clinic treatments. Current medication for other conditions should be noted, especially where drugs may affect the clinician's willingness to perform a nerve block, e.g. anticoagulants.

Psychosocial history

An understanding of the patient's environment is central to understanding the pain. It assesses logistics of domestic and physical support which would be needed for treatments such as day case procedures, the application of transcutaneous electrical nerve stimulation (TENS) machines and coping with the side effects of some drugs.

It looks for psychological aspects of the pain. Psychological assessment begins at the first point of contact and does not require the skills of a psychologist initially. Details of personal, sexual and family relationships, source of income, occupation, ethnic origin and availability of social and psychological support can be sought from the history.

The patient's beliefs about the condition and its progression and expectations of treatment should be asked. Beliefs that imply that the patient is seriously worried about the progression of undiagnosed pathology are 'yellow flags'. Symptoms of anxiety, depression or anger are frequently present and may or may not require therapy. A profile of the patient's activities of daily living and questioning about interpersonal relationships demonstrates behavioural components to pain. Outstanding litigation or compensation claims should be recorded.

Further reading

Bonica JJ. Organization and function of a pain clinic. Advances in Neurology 1974; 4: 433–43.

Related topics of interest

Anatomy and physiology (p. 5); Back pain – medical management (p. 28); Psychosocial assessment of pain (p. 186).

ASSESSMENT OF CHRONIC PAIN – EXAMINATION

This chapter addresses the basics of physical assessment. In other areas of medicine, the physical examination helps to form a diagnosis. In chronic pain the physical assessment has several purposes.

Purpose

1. To exclude conditions better treated by other specialists. Some abnormal physical findings are indications of life-threatening or serious pathology which need to be referred appropriately.

2. To reassure the patient that the pain warrants no further investigation or surgery. This breaks the cycle of repeated investigation without findings to account for pain and unnecessary referral for further medical opinion.

3. To find physical signs associated with pain. Although visceral, neurological and orthopaedic components to pain have been investigated, signs of musculoskeletal tenderness or sensory signs such as allodynia, hyperalgesia and hyperpathia are frequently missed until the pain clinic physician's examination. This may be because the significance of these signs has not been understood.

4. To define baseline signs and monitor changes. All physical signs should be documented at the outset to enable assessment of the effect of treatment or to allow monitoring of deterioration at subsequent physical examination.

5. As a specific search for inconsistencies between symptoms and findings on examination, or during examination in different positions. The presence of inconsistency does not imply 'exaggeration' or 'fraud'. It may simply indicate communication difficulties between different doctors or between doctor and patient. It is a reflection that in chronic pain, amplification of symptoms without obvious findings is to be expected. An example of this is the subjective sensation of swelling that can occur in many painful conditions but may have no objective signs.

Back pain

The back

1. Inspection
- Scars.
- Muscle spasm.
- Structural or postural abnormalities.

2. Palpation
- Spinous processes.
- Area over facet joints.
- Paravertebral areas.

3. Range of movement
- Determination of restriction.
- Attention to provocation of pain: flexion of lumbar spine causing leg pain.
- Rotation or extension of spine provoking pain from posterior structures.

Relevant neurological examination
Neurological examination distinguishes between back pain without root tension signs, back pain with simple root tension signs and back pain with neurological signs which need to be assessed by a surgeon. For thoracic back pain, wasting and sensory abnormalities of the trunk should be excluded. For all back pain, neurological assessment of the legs and perineum should be made as follows:

1. Nerve root tension signs
- Provocation of radicular pain by coughing or sneezing.
- Limited straight-leg raise. Each leg is examined separately. A positive finding on straight leg raise (SLR) is the reproduction of leg or buttock pain. The angle at which this occurs should be noted in degrees. SLR limited by the production of back pain does not necessarily imply nerve root tension. An SLR of less than 10° does not suggest nerve root tension.
- A positive sciatic stretch test is the exacerbation of radicular pain by dorsiflexion of the foot.
- Crossed leg pain is the provocation of pain in the symptomatic leg by straight raising of the other leg. It is highly suggestive of a prolapsed intervertebral disc.
- The finding of apparent tension in one position, e.g. lying, that is not reproduced in the sitting position has been described as an 'inappropriate' sign. The significance of the word 'inappropriate' is in relation to the diagnosis of disc irritation. It is regrettable that this inconsistency has been misinterpreted as implying that the patient is 'misleading' the clinician.

2. Muscle power is assessed by obvious wasting and grading of the following movements:
- Hip flexion dependent on L1 and L2 roots.
- Knee flexion dependent on L5, S1 and S2 roots.
- Knee extension dependent on L3 and L4 roots.
- Ankle plantar flexion dependent on S1 root.
- Ankle dorsiflexion dependent on L4 and L5 roots.
- Extension of the big toe dependent on L5 and S1 roots.

3. Sensation to cotton wool and/or pin prick should be determined according to whether deficiency is in a dermatomal, peripheral nerve or other distribution, such as glove and stocking or whole limb. There may be signs of hyperexcitability such as allodynia, hyperalgesia or hyperpathia.

4. Reflexes. Patellar and ankle reflexes imply intact L3/L4 and S1/S2 nerve roots respectively. Up-going plantars and hyper-reflexia need referral for the investigation of an upper motor neurone problem and lead the examiner to search for a motor, sensory and reflex level.

5. Nerve root signs. Compression of the S1 nerve root by the L5/S1 disc causes weakness of plantar flexion, reduced sensation in the S1 distribution and an absent or diminished ankle jerk. (Symmetrical loss of the ankle jerks is, however, common in the elderly without pathology.) Compression of the L5 nerve root by an L4/L5 disc causes weakness of the extensor hallucis longus, reduced sensation in the L5 distribution but may not result in changes in the reflexes. The findings of paraesthesia of legs and perineum, a lax anal sphincter, weakness of ankle movements with absent ankle reflexes in a patient with back pain requires urgent (same day) exclusion of an acute central disc prolapse, a surgical emergency.

Neck pain

The neck

1. Inspection
- Deformities.
- Scars.
- Muscle atrophy.
- Abnormal vertebral contour.

2. Palpation
- Tenderness.
- Muscle spasm.

3. Range of movement in all parameters
- Determination of restriction.
- Attention to provocation of pain.

Relevant neurological examination

1. Muscle power is assessed by obvious wasting and grading of the following movements:
- Arm abduction dependent on C5 root.
- Elbow flexion dependent on C5 and C6 roots.
- Elbow extension dependent on C7 root.
- Wrist extension dependent on C6 root.
- Wrist flexion dependent on C7 root.
- Finger extension dependent on C7 root.
- Finger flexion and adduction dependent on C8 root.
- Finger abduction dependent on C8 and T1 roots.

2. Sensation is tested in the same way as in the legs during the neurological examination of the back. A common misdiagnosis of a sensory level is when it occurs in the arms – remember that C4 dermatome anteriorly can extend down the chest wall. High sensory level (foramen magnum) can also easily be missed – it occurs along the coronal suture!

3. Reflexes
- Normal biceps reflex implies intact C5 root.
- Normal brachioradialis reflex implies intact C6 root.
- Normal triceps reflex implies intact C7 root.

In cervical myelopathy reflexes may be brisk.

Limb pain

The limb

1. Inspection
- Deformity.
- Wasting.
- Discoloration.
- Oedema or trophic changes, such as loss of hair or shiny skin.

2. Palpation
- Tenderness.
- Muscle spasm.
- Temperature change can be noted by comparison with the opposite limb.

3. Range of movement. Passive and active movement (with quantification of its limitation) estimates function, particularly of a joint.

Head and face pain

Physical examination within the pain clinic is to reinforce that the referral of a face pain or headache is appropriate and does not require other specialist input.

Head and face

1. Inspection
- Face.
- Head.
- Inside of mouth.
- External auditory meatus.

2. Palpation
- Surface of head.
- Temporal arteries.
- Temporomandibular joints for tenderness and clicking on closure, areas of reported tenderness, trigger points or neuromata.
- Facial sinuses.

Relevant neurological examination
- Neuralgias for nerve entrapment causing provocation of pain.
- Trigeminal sensory testing for deficiency and hyperexcitability.
- The presence of 'trigger' points.
- Cranial nerves (corneal reflex, visual fields and acuity, ocular movements), hearing, motor power.

Occlusal analysis
- Interincisal distance should be three finger breadths and closure should be smooth.
- There should be no side-to-side deviation or midline shift as maximum closure is approached.

Abdominal, pelvic and perineal pain

Visceral components of pain presenting to the pain clinic are usually seen by specialists in surgical and medical disciplines prior to referral. Superficial tenderness or sensory abnormality may however not have been noted. It is rarely appropriate to perform a rectal or vaginal examination. If appropriate this should be a chaperoned procedure.

Related topics of interest

Assessment of chronic pain – history (p. 20); Back pain – medical management (p. 34).

BACK PAIN – INJECTIONS

There are several targets for intervention techniques in the treatment of back pain. There are many nerve pathways implicated in the experience of back pain, and as many enthusiasts for one particular technique as there are uncontrolled reports of efficacy. The evidence base for the rational use of injections for back pain is vestigial. The treatment of back pain must be seen in the light of other factors that influence its occurrence and prognosis. Patients with psychological distress or illness behaviour may have unrealistic expectations of treatment. Nerve blocks should be seen as a prerequisite to education and rehabilitation, allowing an opportunity for mobilization and return to normal activity.

This discussion will consider several aspects of spinal injection practice:

- Injections around the facet joints.
- Destruction of spinal nerves.
- Epidural steroid injections.
- Epidural and nerve root injections: advanced techniques.

Anatomy

Posterior structures of the motion segment are innervated by the dorsal primary ramus of the spinal nerve. The structures are:

- Facet joints.
- Posterior part of the dura.
- Ligaments.
- Back muscles.

Anterior structures are innervated by a nerve plexus (the sinuvertebral nerve) which enters the spinal nerve in the sympathetic communicating ramus and projects to several levels of the spinal cord. The structures are:

- Vertebral bodies.
- Longitudinal ligaments.
- Discs.
- Anterior part of the dura.
- Paravertebral muscles.

Nerve blocks in diagnosis and treatment

Block of the medial branch of the dorsal primary ramus of the spinal nerve may confirm a diagnosis of pain from the posterior elements of the motion segment. Theoretically, blocks of the sinuvertebral nerve may help to confirm the diagnosis of pain from the anterior elements. In practice, however, only the former approach can localize the anatomical area responsible, as the projections of the sinuvertebral nerve cover several vertebral levels. Provocative discography – injection into the intervertebral disc with the aim of identifying a source of pain – may be valuable for localizing an anterior source of pain. The anatomical segmental localization of posterior element pain by selective injection is confounded by variable contributions to the facet joints from segments above and below, but the procedure is nevertheless valuable in confirming a clinical suspicion of posterior element pain and is an essential prerequisite for nerve destruction techniques.

Techniques

Injections around the facet joints

Two techniques that have to be considered are:

- The use of local anaesthetic with or without steroid in or around the facet joint.
- The use of local anaesthetic to identify a sensory nerve pathway responsible for pain with the aim of destroying it.

The lumbar facet joints are easily accessible for both techniques and are served by a specific nerve supply that has little in the way of cutaneous representation. Although the injections may be considered by the casual observer, and the patient, to be similar procedures, they are in fact different in respect of the target for injection and the rationale for the procedure. The former is an attempt to treat the joint itself, the latter is an attempt to interrupt the pain pathways from the joint. Such diversity of rationale has hampered the quest for evidence for efficacy for these injections, as experts have their own techniques. The actual technique of injection may vary between clinicians and may be accomplished with varying degrees of difficulty depending upon the radiological appearance. Whereas the 'gold standard' for injection is the accurate placement of a low volume of anaesthetic within the joint or on the medial branch of the segmental posterior primary ramus, it may be difficult or impossible to achieve, and anaesthetic may, instead, be deposited on adjacent paravertebral tissues and somatic nerve roots, leading to a clinical effect that may be falsely attributed to facet joint involvement.

Controlled trials have noted that there is a placebo effect from lumbar facet joint injection. This has led to the recommendation that the procedure be undertaken on two separate occasions, using local anaesthetic of different duration (e.g. lidocaine and bupivacaine) with the intention of demonstrating that the drug with the longer pharmacological effect has a longer clinical duration. In practice, this is often difficult to demonstrate, and an alternative explanation has to be found for patients who report pain relief that far outlasts the pharmacological action of a drug. Explanations include the reduction of muscle spasm with facilitation of painless movement under the influence of the block or the effects of a short-lasting peripheral anaesthetic block on central processing, and of course, the placebo effect.

Investigators have used many different techniques to study the effect of facet joint steroid injection. A systematic review identified four prospective trials.

One of these showed that the accurate placement of steroid within the facet joint (as opposed to around the joint) was important for pain relief. Another study, on a population of patients who had previously responded to facet joint local anaesthetic injections, showed that the benefits of steroids were short lived. This latter observation is of clear relevance to the clinician: in practice it is difficult to refuse repeated injections for the patient who reports improvement of mobility and reduction of pain symptoms for a few weeks. It is important that when such procedures are used, the patient and clinician are aware of the time limitations, the potential dangers of repeated X-ray exposure and steroid administration, and the possibility of the patient adopting a purely 'passive' approach to the long-term management of the problem.

Destruction of spinal nerves

The safe execution of nerve destruction (neurotomy) techniques has a few prerequisites:

- The nerve pathway has been identified by a trial local anaesthetic block.
- The anatomy (and its variations) of the target nerve is clearly understood.
- The target nerve has insignificant cutaneous distribution.
- The target nerve has insignificant motor function.
- The radiological anatomy can be clearly demonstrated – it is helpful if the nerve is located close to a bony radiological landmark.
- There is minimal risk of damage to surrounding structures.

Neurotomy can be achieved with chemical, radiofrequency current (high temperature or normal temperature) or cryotherapy techniques. Radiofrequency current techniques are well described for the lumbar spine: the medial branch of the primary dorsal ramus of the lumbar segmental nerve fulfils all the prerequisites above. (In the cervical spine, however, the proximity of the vertebral artery is a potential danger for the high temperature technique.) The nerve can be located easily by reference to radiological landmarks (the eye of the 'Scotty dog' on oblique projection of the lumbar vertebra). Trial electrical stimulation at low voltage is used to position the needle close to the nerve and to ensure that the needle tip is away from the mixed nerve root.

Systematic review has identified four small prospective trials of the efficacy of high-temperature radiofrequency lesioning, all of which supported the technique. The effectiveness of the technique over a period of 12 months was noted in two studies. As well as a reduction of pain, as measured with a visual analogue scale, one investigator has shown an improvement in disability rating scales. It is of considerable interest that success for the technique has been claimed when symptoms have been present for many years, and, in respect of one study of the technique used on the cervical spine, successful pain relief is claimed to be associated with resolution of psychological distress.

A number of neurotomy techniques are also used for spinal nerves other than the medial branch of the dorsal ramus described above. These techniques are limited by the relative proximity of other structures, and the multiple functions served by the nerves. A hierarchy of techniques, progressing from the lowest risk, simplest technique is therefore proposed The technique chosen will be determined by the probable diagnosis supported by appropriate diagnostic local anaesthetic tests and competence and experience of the operator. The hierarchy has been described as (in increasing order of technical difficulty):

- Facet joint lesion (medial branch of primary dorsal ramus).
- Lumbar sympathetic chain lesion.
- Lumbar disc lesion.
- Lesion of the communicating ramus.
- Lesion of the dorsal root ganglion.

Lumbar sympathetic chain and communicating ramus lesions have been described for pain which involves the pathways of the sympathetic system and sinuvertebral nerve. This is pain from the anterior structures of the spine, again assessed by history and the response to local anaesthetic block.

The same nerve pathways may be lesioned in lumbar disc lesions. In this technique, the radiofrequency probe is inserted into the disc. The thermal conductivity of the disc material and the lack of vascularity to the disc results in a gradient of temperature across the disc, with an effect on the nociceptors of the annulus fibrosus.

The dorsal root ganglion contains the cell bodies of primary afferent nociceptors and of larger, faster-conducting fibres serving modalities of touch and vibration sense. The technique of dorsal root ganglion lesion carries with it the risk of causing damage to these latter neurones, resulting in anaesthesia of the skin. This risk is reduced by the use of a lower temperature for lesioning fibres, thereby causing a selective action on the unmyelinated small nociceptor neurones. A specific technique that allows this lower-temperature lesion is pulsed radiofrequency current.

Epidural steroid injections

The rationale for the use of steroids in the epidural space is the presence of inflammation around nerve roots. Many reports and observational studies claiming benefit for epidural steroids predated systematic study with controlled trials. Two systematic reviews are reported here. One has found six randomized controlled trials supporting the use of epidural steroids for the short-term treatment of back pain with leg pain, and an equal number of trials failing to conclude the same. By pooling results from randomized controlled trials, a second review has calculated number needed to treat (NNT) of epidural steroids of 7 for 75% pain relief at 60 days and 13 for 50% pain relief at 1 year. There is controversy surrounding the use of epidural steroids, however, not least in view of some of the claims that have been made for them, and for intrathecal steroids. Historically, epidural and intrathecal steroids have been used for a number of conditions, and recently suggested in the management of postherpetic neuralgia. In common with many drugs used by pain clinicians, depot steroids do not have a product licence for epidural use. Indeed, advice has been given in the past that epidural steroids, even correctly administered, should not be used because of neurotoxicity. (This advice was based on anecdotal Australian reports that were never substantiated.) One manufacturer actively discourages the practice of epidural injection by printing warnings on the ampoule. Of concern is the presence of benzyl alcohol and/or polyethylene glycol, a non-ionic detergent in the pharmaceutical preparation. The risk of accidental administration into the subarachnoid space should be considered: methylprednisolone can cause arachnoiditis if so injected. Every effort should be made to ensure that the drug is deposited outside the dura. As with facet joint injections, there is no consensus on the practice of repeated epidural injections for relapsing symptoms. It is difficult to deny any patient who derives relief for a number of weeks the chance of having the procedure repeated. The possibility of a cumulative effect of repeated steroid administration is one factor that may influence practice.

Paravertebral and dorsal root ganglion injections are variants of the epidural steroid injection, targeting specific nerve roots, and should be considered identical in respect of the risks of steroid administration, cardiovascular and intrathecal injection. Specific indications for these blocks include unilateral symptoms, evidence of a single level of lesion responsible for the pain and symptoms from nerve compression/irritation in the lateral foramen.

Epidural and nerve root injections: advanced techniques

The use of a radiographic contrast medium in the epidural space can demonstrate anatomical variants and scar tissue around the nerves of the cauda equina after spinal surgery, and as a natural consequence of the inflammatory response to leakage of disc material from degenerate intervertebral discs. The technique enables the operator to observe the nerve root during injection of drugs into the epidural space and to target the drug to the radiological lesion and free the nerve from scar tissue by a hydrostatic pressure effect. The use of saline, local anaesthetic, steroids, hyaluronidase and hypertonic saline under X-ray guidance has been reported. A refinement of the technique involves the introduction of a fine catheter or spinal endoscope into the epidural space with the aim of drug delivery near the site of radicular symptoms and direct visualization of the response to attempted hydrostatic distension and adhesiolysis of nerve roots.

There are now data from controlled studies that help to put this latter therapy into context. In patients with short-term symptoms (less than 10 months) of sciatica and no history of spinal surgery, there would appear to be no advantage in using spinal endoscopy to place the steroid accurately within the spinal canal. However, with more chronic radicular symptoms, after failure of conventional epidural injection or after surgery, endoscopic visualization with hydrostatic distension of scarred nerve roots provides better pain relief than endoscopic steroid administration alone.

Systematic reviews

Koes BW, Scholten RJPM, Mens JMA, Bouter LM. Efficacy of epidural steroid injections for low back pain and sciatica: a systematic review of randomized clinical trials. Pain 1995; 63: 279–88.

Slipman CW, Bhat AL, Gilchrist RV, et al. A critical review of the evidence for the use of zygoapophysial injections and radiofrequency denervation in the treatment of low back pain. The Spine Journal 2003; 3: 310–16

Watts RW, Silagy CA. A meta-analysis on the efficacy of epidural corticosteroids in the treatment of sciatica. Anaesthesia and Intensive Care 1994; 23: 564–9.

Further reading

Manchikanti L, Boswell MV, Rivera RJ, et al. A randomized, controlled trial of spinal endoscopic adhesiolysis in chronic refractory low back and lower extremity pain. BMC Anesthesiol 2005, 5: 10.

Stolker RJ, Vervest ACM, Groen GJ. The management of chronic spinal pain by blockades: a review. Pain 1994; 58: 1–20.

Related topics of interest

Back pain – medical management (p. 28); Nerve blocks and therapeutic lesions – general principles (p. 104).

BACK PAIN – MEDICAL MANAGEMENT

Low back pain currently accounts for more than half of all musculoskeletal disability, whereas work loss due to back pain in the UK is approximately 52 million days per year. Disability due to low back pain has reached epidemic proportions, although there is no evidence for an increase in pathology. The cost of treating back pain is 1% of the total UK NHS budget. Assessment of the back pain sufferer establishes:

- Whether there is serious or systemic disease.
- Whether there is nerve root involvement.
- The presence, by exclusion, of the condition known as chronic mechanical back pain

It is intended that this assessment be carried out in the acute stage of initial presentation and at regular intervals thereafter. In many cases the diagnosis of non-specific low back pain can be made with confidence. Once this clinical diagnosis has been achieved, further investigation is not required, unless there is a significant change in the pain.

Serious or systemic disease

The following factors should alert to the possibility of serious or systemic disease. Features are referred to as 'red flags'. The reporting of such a symptom is a 'red flag' for the presence of a serious condition that needs investigation.

1. Symptoms of serious disease
- Bilateral or alternating symptoms.
- Constant or progressive pain.
- Night-time pain.
- Morning stiffness, relieved by exercise.
- Acute onset in the elderly.
- History of cancer.
- Fever or night sweats.
- Immunosuppression.
- Recent bacterial infection.
- Acute neurological symptoms, such as painful footdrop, perineal sensory impairment or sphincter disturbance.

2. Examination
- Tenderness on sacroiliac springing.
- Multiple nerve root signs suggesting compression over a number of lumbar segments from tumour or dissociative signs suggestive of intrinsic cord pathology.
- Symmetrical limitation of straight leg raising.
- Spinal rigidity, tenderness or deformity such as kyphus or step.
- Absent lower limb pulses or other features of lower limb ischaemia.
- Abdominal mass.

In the presence of red flags the following conditions should be considered as possible causes of back pain. The list is not exhaustive, but further discussion on the investigation of these conditions is not within the scope of this text:

- Aortic aneurysm.
- Retroperitoneal fibrosis.
- Tumour (primary or secondary).
- Gynaecological pathology.
- Ankylosing spondylitis.
- Metabolic bone disease.
- Infection.
- Osteoporosis.
- Paget's disease.
- Pott's disease.
- Myeloma.

Simple investigations such as erythrocyte sedimentation rate (ESR), blood count, bone biochemistry, lumbar spine and sacroiliac joint X-ray or isotope bone scan can be easily organized before referral is made for definitive management.

Back pain with nerve root involvement

With the proviso that the acute presentation of the cauda equina syndrome of perineal numbness, bilateral leg pain and sphincter disturbance described above is recognized as a 'red flag' necessitating immediate surgical referral, other nerve root problems in the absence of 'red flags' can be treated symptomatically. Nerve root involvement may be treatable surgically. It is said that symptoms differ depending on whether nerve roots are irritated or compressed by disc or bony stenosis, being experienced as pain or numbness, respectively. As a general rule, decompression is said to be more likely to be successful if it is carried out before the onset of numbness, which may be a late feature. Symptoms result from compression or irritation of the nerve root by either disc, bone or ligamentous hypertrophy. Symptoms and signs are of numbness and weakness in the appropriate dermatome and myotome, with loss of reflex at the corresponding root level and pain in the dermatome made worse by the manoeuvre of the sciatic or femoral stretch test.

Compression of the nerve root by a far lateral disc protrusion in the lateral foramen may cause diagnostic confusion with a high lumbar disc prolapse, with pain referred to the front of the thigh. However, the far lateral disc lesion may also be associated with muscle wasting due to direct compression of motor nerve roots that allows the differential diagnosis to be made on clinical grounds. Neurogenic claudication (pain on walking associated with spinal stenosis) may be confused with intermittent claudication of vascular origin, but distinguished from it by its slower recovery course and radicular distribution.

Non-specific low back pain

The diagnosis of non-specific or 'idiopathic' low back pain is one of exclusion. The diagnosis must be considered in the wider context of functional and psychosocial limitation, with an overall aim of reducing the disability as well as controlling symptoms.

If a diagnosis of non-specific low back pain is entertained, further observations may be valuable in defining an anatomical origin. However, the search for relevant pathology may be fruitless. Although magnetic resonance imaging (MRI) is a non-invasive and safe way of investigating back pain, the sensitivity of this technique is such that a distressed patient will focus on minor and incidental abnormalities that are not responsible for the symptoms. MRI demonstrates minor abnormalities of the intervertebral disc in up to 30% of asymptomatic subjects. Furthermore, it has been elegantly shown that while the precision of diagnosis may be helped by such investigation, management by the clinician requesting the examination does not change as a consequence of the refined diagnosis. Attempts at rehabilitation should not await the completion of such investigation. The clinician must understand that the decision to investigate carries with it the risk of undermining the patient's confidence in the clinical diagnosis. It may reinforce a false belief that there is something seriously wrong. Prior discussion with a radiologist who understands the clinical significance of this may avoid the danger of making too much of the presence of inconsequential scan findings. Conversely, it has also been demonstrated that a scan that is undertaken to 'reassure' a patient and is reported as normal will worsen distress and also undermine the confidence between patient and professional. The solution is to limit the use of MRI to those cases where there is suspicion of pathology or where a particular intervention requiring a precise anatomical diagnosis is required.

The site of the pain may be defined in terms of symptoms in two different ways: one way seeks to identify the anatomical location responsible according to symptoms, the other describes the spine as a series of segments. Both models have their uses in diagnosis and treatment.

Specific anatomical syndromes

The suggestion that radiological changes in the lumbar zygoapophyseal (facet) joints indicate a cause for the pain was first entertained in 1911, but there is no correlation between the X-ray appearance and the degree of pain. The idea of a specific 'facet syndrome' as a clinical diagnosis is by no means universally accepted. Where it is used, however, it relates to a symptom complex that describes pain from the posterior structures of the vertebral column, and to be compared with other diagnoses.

1. Facet syndrome
- Continuous pain.
- Worsened by rotation and extension.
- Radiation into the leg or the gluteal area, in a dermatomal or non-dermatomal distribution.
- Tenderness over the joints and paravertebral muscle spasm.

2. Ligamentous pain
- Pain worsened by flexion and extension.
- Tenderness is worse when the back muscles are relaxed.

3. Pain from vertebral body
- Back pain radiating to buttock and leg.
- Straight leg raising worsens the back pain but not the leg pain.

4. Pain from sacroiliac joints
- Buttock and leg pain worsen immediately on weight bearing.

Lumbar segmental dysfunction

This concept considers that the spine is a series of bony segments connected by motion segments. Each motion segment therefore consists of part of the body of adjacent vertebrae, the intervertebral disc, the paired zygoapophyseal joints and the associated ligaments, capsules and muscles and fascia. All these structures have nociceptors, except for the nucleus pulposus and the inner two-thirds of the annulus fibrosus, and therefore have the potential to be a site of origin of pain. The concept is a useful alternative to a fruitless search for non-existent pathology in the anatomical structures.

Lumbar segmental dysfunction is defined as lumbar pain, ostensibly due to excessive strains imposed on the restraining elements of a single spinal motion segment. The clinical features of lumbar segmental dysfunction are lumbar spinal pain, with or without referred pain that can be aggravated by selectively stressing a particular spinal motion segment. There is tenderness detectable locally and also at a distance in the areas of referred pain. Diagnostic confusion may be caused if it is not realized that autonomic changes may also occur.

Diagnostic criteria. All the following criteria should be satisfied:

- The affected motion segment must be specified.
- Pain is aggravated by clinical tests that selectively stress the affected motion segment.
- Stressing adjacent motion segments does not reproduce the patient's pain.

The diagnosis of segmental dysfunction is one step in establishing a possible site of origin of spinal pain. Because the innervation of a particular motion segment may be from more than one nerve, and because primary nociceptive fibres project widely onto spinal cord neurones, identification of a single lumbar segmental dysfunction may be difficult.

In practice the two concepts can be combined. Blocks of the medial branch of the dorsal primary ramus of the spinal segmental nerve spine, or the sinu-vertebral nerve, may refine the diagnosis to the painful structure to posterior or anterior elements of the spine, respectively. Further investigations, such as the injection of radiographic contrast medium into the intervertebral disc or the synovial cavity of a facet joint, might help refine the diagnosis.

Management of acute and chronic back pain

The optimum management of 'idiopathic' back pain thus remains a controversial issue. It is clear that there is no one 'correct' way of treating the symptoms. In practice many patients will be prescribed paracetamol/codeine preparations, anti-inflammatory drugs, and some will claim that opioids alone provide sufficient relief for normal activity to be undertaken. Decisions to use drugs licensed for neuropathic pain may also be made in the belief that buttock or leg pain is due to nerve root irritation, when precise anatomical diagnosis is difficult.

Using many different treatment modalities (ice, local heat, transcutaneous nerve stimulation, interferential, traction, mobilization, etc.), physiotherapy has been largely unsuccessful in providing long-term relief of symptoms, although individual therapists are keen to use techniques that work in their hands, if only for short periods of time. Indeed, it is now seen that the aim of treatment as one of providing long-term relief of pain is unrealistic and that the purpose of therapy is preventing the progression of pain to immobility and disability that is a consequence of fear of movement. The key to successful management is one of looking at the symptoms within a broader context of reduction of disability and tackling beliefs about the nature and significance of the spinal pain. This requires a multidisciplinary approach with a uniform and agreed strategy for imparting diagnostic information, the avoidance of ambiguous terms to describe irrelevant pathology and an approach that requires the patient to take responsibility for his or her own management. Of the various attempts to draw conclusions from reviews of well-conducted trials, one result is of particular importance in the management of back pain.

Bed rest delays recovery and return to work in acute back ache. Patients who stay in bed report no less pain at later follow up compared with those who stay active. It is no better to stay in bed for 7 days than it is for 2–3 days.

How is such a philosophy – that back pain is not 'curable' in a conventional sense – compatible with some of the published evidence of the short- and intermediate-term benefits of techniques such as nerve block and nerve destruction? The apparent discrepancy can be understood in terms of the complexity of nociceptive inputs involved: discs, joints, ligaments, muscles, nerve roots, spinal cord and brain, and also in respect of the very powerful influence that emotions and beliefs have on the ability to remain active. The concept of the pain presenting a 'moving target' to the clinician as the source of it 'migrates' into the central nervous system progressively with time is a valuable one. It explains the many frustrations of attempting to provide long-term relief by attending solely to presumed peripheral pathology.

Further reading

Back Pain. Report of a CSAG Committee on Back Pain (Chaired by M. Rosen). London: HMSO, 1994.

Cohen JE, Goel V, Frank JW, et al. Group education interventions for people with low back pain. An overview of the literature. Spine 1994; 19: 1214–22.

Gillan MCG, Gilbert FJ, Andrew JE, et al. Influence of Imaging on Clinical Decision making in the Treatment of Lower Back Pain. Radiology 2001; 220: 393–9.

Systematic reviews

Evans G, Richards S. Low back pain: an evaluation of therapeutic interventions. University of Bristol, Health Care Evaluation Unit; p. 176.

Koes BW, Vantulder MW, Vanderwindt DAWM, Bouter LM. The efficacy of back schools: a review of randomised clinical trials. Journal of Clinical Epidemiology 1994; 47: 851–2.

Turner JA, Denny MC. Do antidepressant medications relieve chronic low back pain? Journal of Family Practice 1993; 37: 545–53.

Related topics of interest

Assessment of chronic pain – history (p. 13); Back pain – injections (p. 28); Back pain – surgery (p. 40); Musculoskeletal pain syndromes (p. 95); Psychosocial assessment (p. 181); Therapy – anti-inflammatory drugs (p. 211).

BACK PAIN – SURGERY

This chapter is intended as a brief review of spinal surgery; it consists of an account of two categories of condition: those which constitute the majority of the practice of spinal surgery and a number of other conditions which, though rare, present with axial pain. Being rare, the evidence for the management of such conditions is largely anecdotal, and based on basic surgical principles. As it is an immense subject in its own right, the problems of rheumatoid arthritis, ankylosing spondylitis and scoliosis are not mentioned here.

Lumbar disc disease

The vast majority of spinal surgery is performed for lumbar disc prolapse. The incidence of lumbar disc degeneration is so high as to consider it a normal part of the ageing process. Often it will be asymptomatic, even when prolapse has occurred. In post-mortem studies of asymptomatic individuals, the rate of prolapse is 15%. MRI scans cannot therefore be relied on to make a diagnosis of symptomatic anatomical abnormality, and much trouble ensues if the patient is made aware of normal degenerative changes without being made aware of their lack of clinical significance. Disc disease may present with either or both of low back pain or radicular symptoms. The former is due to the direct damage to the disc, whereas the latter to the effects of the disc protrusion itself. Low back pain is discussed elsewhere but suffice it to mention it may arise from sources other than the disc, such as the muscles, ligaments, facet joints or the dural tube itself – this is not an exhaustive list.

Disc prolapse

These may be considered to be contained or sequestered. The latter means that the nucleus of the disc has burst through the annulus. The earliest description of surgery for disc disease was by Dandy in 1921 (readers will remember he also first described microvascular decompression for trigeminal neuralgia), though the paper of Mixter and Barr in 1934 launched disc surgery.

'Typical'

The most common presentation of disc prolapse is radicular pain, i.e. sciatica. It may be preceded by a back strain or injury; and with an initial acute low back pain which settles to be replaced by sciatica. If the pain radiates below the knee in a dermatomal distribution, then it is highly likely to be radicular in origin, though this is not an absolute rule. It is often associated with motor and sensory deficit relevant to the level of the prolapse; there should be root tension signs such as limitation of straight leg raise. 95% of disc prolapse occurs at L4/5 or L5/S1 and the presenting signs will give some indication of the level although not reliably enough to confirm the level for a surgical approach.

Central

One of two variants of the presentation of lumbar disc prolapse, important because of its dire neurological consequences if missed, a central disc prolapse results in neurological deficit in the cauda equina, which may cause loss of function of bowel control, bladder control and sexual function. Saddle anaesthesia is typical, and sufficient nerves may be affected to result in lower motor neurone weakness of the lower limbs and hence difficulty in walking in addition to the effects of the pain. Pain is usual, and may include sciatic elements as well as the central cauda equina features. Disc decompression must be undertaken as an emergency. With this condition and with the more usual disc prolapse the contribution of lumbar spinal stenosis may be as significant as the disc prolapse itself. The prognosis for recovery of function – bladder, bowel and sexual – following central disc prolapse is much poorer than generally appreciated, even with prompt surgery. Some loss of function is common, and poorly reported by the patient.

Far lateral

This syndrome is becoming increasingly recognized with the advent of cross-sectional imaging, in particular magnetic resonance imaging (MRI). The disc prolapse is outside the spinal canal – truly 'far lateral'. There may be a previous history of back injury, and complaint is of sharp back pain followed by pain in the hip and the anterior thigh. There may be associated weakness of the quadriceps. Its recognition is important: firstly so as not to miss structural pathology as a cause of the low pain and secondly as the surgical approach is different – unsurprisingly it is usually lateral!

Investigations

In virtually all situations this is by MRI, though occasionally myelography, usually with computed tomography (CT) assistance, is required. One obvious indication is when the patient is intolerant of MRI due to claustrophobia; otherwise, it may be used when clinical history and signs convince the clinician but the imaging does not! This reflects the fact that there are no good studies validating myelography – the previous standard – against MRI. The impact of non-invasive imaging is so as to render the role of examination of the patient more to confirm the clinical meaning of the findings on imaging than to attempt precise diagnosis of level or process.

Treatment

It should not be forgotten that the natural history of sciatica due to disc prolapse is for it to resolve, although this may take some considerable time. In one study it has been claimed that there was no difference in symptoms of sciatica 10 years after surgery comparing an operated with a non-operated group. One further interesting statistic is that the rate of operation for lumbar disc surgery is 100/100 000 in the UK but this rises to 900/100 000 in the USA where there is abundant provision of the facilities for the investigation and surgical treatment of this condition. However, 90% of attacks of sciatica will settle conservatively; if a second attack occurs then the likelihood of remaining attack-free in the future falls to 50% and is further reduced with subsequent attacks. The risk of recurrent attacks also increases if the protrusion is not contained. Thus, there is some evidence to confirm the clinical impression of neurosurgeons that large sequestered disc prolapses do cause recurrent severe episodes of sciatica, do well surgically, and that patients should therefore be advised with confidence that microdiscectomy is currently the best option.

The gold standard for treatment is microdiscectomy and is effective in over 90% in providing relief of sciatica. In perhaps 50% of cases back pain will be improved. The results are less good when recovery of neurological function is considered. This is important when the cauda equina is at risk, but the impact of a persistent foot drop should not be underestimated. The chance of recovery depends on the time for which function has been lost and this is why decompression for central disc is performed as an emergency. It is said that the chance of neurological recovery is better when pain is still present.

The operative philosophy is to minimize structural damage to the spine, so a unilateral muscle strip is performed and a small fenestration made in the interlaminar space. The success rate is related to the degree of prolapse and those patients with 'negative explorations' do poorly. The use of the microscope has been associated with reduced hospital stay, and less denervation of paraspinal muscles when compared to open procedures, though an open procedure with full laminectomy may be necessary to provide safe access to large central disc protrusions. Occasionally the only way to obtain safe access to a central lumbar disc prolapse may be to go transdurally and remove a fragment by separating the nerves of the cauda equina. A popular patient misconception is that the whole disc is removed – in fact only the part containing the protrusion is removed with perhaps some further amount from the disc space. Disc weights indicate that the average volume of disc removed is only 6–8% of the total. Surgery does not come without risk. There is a mortality rate (though low) due to thromboembolism, but there may also be infection including discitis. Epidural fibrosis may be one of the causes, not the only one, for a chronic pain state – the failed back syndrome. Other treatments have been attempted for contained disc prolapse including chymopapain injection, percutaneous nucleotomy and laser microdiscectomy. None of these have found wide acceptance; in the case of percutaneous nucleotomy, a prospective randomized controlled trial showed it to be inferior to microdiscectomy. Chymopapain is dangerous if mistakenly injected into the subarachnoid space. There are no controlled randomized data regarding laser treatments as shown by its failure to gain acceptance.

Neurogenic claudication and lumbar spinal stenosis

As the name suggests this presents as pain made worse on walking. Typically the pain is radicular, and takes about 10–15 min to resolve. These two features distinguish it from arterial claudication. Examination in the clinic is often normal, again in contrast to arterial claudication. One feature of the history that is occasionally mentioned is that symptoms improve as the patient bends forward, for example to rest on a neighbour's garden gate after a fixed walking distance.

Investigation is by MRI, though if this fails then CT myelography may be used. The natural history is for the condition to be relatively stable so that conservative treatment after making the diagnosis is adequate. The conventional surgical treatment is by laminectomy and decompression though recently there is a trend to more conservative operations – multilevel fenestrations and undercutting facetectomy. This is because of the fear of destabilizing the back, though in practice this seldom happens.

In exceptional circumstances medical treatment may be required. This is not as effective as the surgical treatment and is reserved for patients unfit for surgery, or those unwilling to accept surgery. The anticonvulsants may be tried – sodium valproate or carbamazepine or as an alternative calcitonin. Variably these attempts may produce success for a year or so.

Low back pain

Critical analysis of surgery for low back pain in the context of degenerative disease is not encouraging. By contrast, indications for instrumentation, fusion and stabilization in cases of trauma, tumour, deformity or severe spondylolisthesis are accepted. Since this is a surgical chapter no reference is made to the psychological aspects of the problem except to note that these are of great importance – and dealt with elsewhere in this book.

When discectomy is performed purely for back pain the results are not good. There is much written regarding the role of spinal fusion with or without concomitant stabilization, and many major operations have been carried out for back pain on the basis that this is due to an 'unstable' back, which can therefore be corrected by spinal stabilization. There is much energy invested in the design and production of different types of instrumentation, and in addition image-guided fluoroscopic techniques for safe placement of said instrumentation. However, randomized trials, which are few in number and often methodologically flawed, have not demonstrated any benefit from such operations compared with best physical therapy and the popularity has therefore declined for such procedures in the UK though in North America the practice continues. For example in one study although fusion resulted in some improvement compared with control, the treatment group included an active rehabilitation regimen so that it was unclear whether the surgery or this regimen produced the benefit. Again, as with disc surgery, the operation rate is much higher in the USA than in UK, at 80 compared with 15 per 100 000, respectively. If it is assumed that the spectrum of pathology is broadly similar, then widely differing sets of indications for surgery must exist.

Trials of intradiscal electrotherapy for back pain have demonstrated no benefit over placebo for this technique, which can no longer be recommended. Since the method seems to amount to a disc denervation procedure, previous experience of procedures for pain relief would not lead to optimism as to the outcome of such a trial.

The joints in the vertebral column are complex, so one problem has always been to make a diagnosis as to which structure might be responsible for the pain. Proper sensitivity and specificity analyses for diagnostic tests – which comprise either provocation techniques such as discography or local anaesthetic blocks such as facet joint injections – have never been presented. More recently, fMRI data from group analyses suggested that the origin of the pain may be more in the central and affective components of the pain matrix, which is in keeping with the failure of interventional procedures, difficulties in identifying a structural cause for the pain and the known psychological influences on pain in this situation. These remarks apply also to failed back surgery syndrome – perhaps with even more force (see below). Thus the failure of primarily physical treatments should not in fact be a surprise.

There continues to be interest in the use of spinal cord stimulation for low back pain. It is frequently observed that in cases stimulated for leg pain – usually failed back syndrome – the associated low back pain improves also. However, despite enthusiasm, this indication lacks proof of efficacy, though advances in spinal cord stimulation methodology may alter this situation. Intrathecal drug delivery systems using opioids are reported to have some successes.

Spondylolisthesis

This describes the situation where there is forward slip of one vertebra on another. In many instances it is asymptomatic but when it presents it is usually with back pain. The back pain is aggravated by activity and relieved by rest. The slip may also cause nerve root compression and therefore leg pain. Occasionally fusion is advised – principally in a younger age group (<35 years) – but usually conservative treatment is the rule, contact sports being avoided in the young age group. Decompression of the nerve root is helpful for leg pain, especially in patients over the age of 35 years in whom progression of slip is unlikely. This can be done by a 'microdisc' approach.

Failed back surgery syndrome

Failed back surgery syndrome is an emotive expression describing the situation where there is persistence of symptoms following low back surgery. The incidence is about 5–10%. Of these, perhaps as many as 15% may represent recurrent disc prolapse, and 50–60% may be due to unrecognized lateral recess stenosis. Perhaps 20% are due to epidural fibrosis or arachnoiditis, and it is these cases that are of interest to the pain clinician and may be considered to be a variety of neuropathic pain. (It is worth noting that these cases may respond well to spinal cord stimulation, especially where leg pain is the predominant feature.) Clearly the high incidence of structural and surgically remediable problems requires thorough investigation by imaging of failed back cases, and consideration for surgery. One difficult situation is where there is a combination of fibrosis and disc recurrence. Even with modern imaging it can be difficult to resolve this dilemma. However, the results of reoperation have been shown to be worse than those of spinal cord stimulation.

Thoracic disc

This is a very rare syndrome, with an incidence of only 1/1 000 000. Presenting features are back pain, radicular pain in an intercostal distribution and thoracic myelopathy. However pain is not the predominant feature and signs and symptoms of myelopathy are more common. Surgical excision is the treatment and this may involve a transthoracic approach.

Tumours

Intrinsic cord lesions

Intrinsic tumours of the spinal cord are rare; presentation is by neurological deficit in the main, though a dull aching axial pain is often present. Because of the rarity of the condition diagnosis is often made after a delay. Occasionally (and see also syringomyelia) the neurological deficit may involve insensitivity to pain. Some tumours may be associated with central cord cysts, and this situation is sometimes classified as a type of syringomyelia. Management of the tumours is by biopsy and if possible surgical resection; occasionally this resection may be followed by central spinal cord neuropathic pain. Depending on the histology radiotherapy or chemotherapy may be offered.

Extrinsic cord lesions

In the region of the conus, lesions such as ependymoma or neurofibroma cause a continuous and progressive pain. Clinically the pain is out of proportion to the signs and demeanour of the patient. Patients may get the label of exhibiting abnormal illness behaviour because of the distress and the lack of corresponding clinical signs. Such conditions can only be diagnosed by imaging, but it is important that the patient is aware of the indication for this. It is important to have an understanding that if investigation fails to demonstrate pathology subsequent treatment should be aimed at the distress and behaviour.

Meningioma, typically found in middle-aged women in the mid-thoracic zone, rarely presents with pain, typical findings being progressive paraparesis.

Tumours of the spinal column

Apart from extremely rare primary bone tumours most lesions are metastatic. Pain may be of two types, with different treatment consequences. Instability pain arises when bone destruction by the metastasis renders the spine mechanically unstable. Pain is worse on movement, and refractory to analgesics whatever their potency. In these circumstances spinal fixation may be indicated. Secondly the pain may be continuous and represent the direct effect of the tumour; in this situation it is usually steroid responsive in the short-term and radiotherapy is effective. In recent years this presentation of metastatic tumour has become much rarer perhaps due to earlier detection by imaging and treatment by radiotherapy. However a recent randomized controlled trial of surgery and radiotherapy versus surgery found significantly in favour of the surgical group, both in terms of survival, ambulation and pain relief, so a more aggressive approach to surgery is indicated. Another technique useful for this group of patients, and which has also been applied to osteoporotic collapse, is percutaneous vertebroplasty. Bone cement is injected into the affected vertebral body percutaneously via the pedicle under fluoroscopic guidance. If there is spinal cord compression by tumour the technique is relatively contraindicated, but results of the technique are good.

Syrinx

A cavity in the spinal cord which may be as a result of tumour, trauma or Arnold–Chiari malformation. It is one of a number of conditions that may cause central spinal cord pain – a situation analogous to central post-stroke pain. Although treatment of the syrinx (shunting or third ventriculostomy for hydrocephalus, hind brain decompression or direct shunting of the syrinx itself) is necessary to prevent disease progression, pain is rarely relieved. Treatment must then be medical, but this is a difficult pain condition to manage.

Miscellaneous conditions

A number of infections may present with spinal pain. All are rare in the UK. **Acute pyogenic infection**, usually causing epidural abscess, causes severe local spinal pain, and the severity of the pain may suggest this diagnosis. Pain from tuberculosis is less acute and is more often related to instability due to the destructive nature of the condition.

Herpes zoster may present with spinal and dermatomal pain. Although the diagnosis is easy to make once vesicles have appeared in a segmental distribution, it may be missed before this feature has appeared.

Spinal subarachnoid haemorrhage occurs but is very rare. It can be due to spinal arteriovenous malformation (AVM) and this may have associated aneurysms. It presents with ictus, and in addition to spinal pain there may be radicular pain and meningism. Interestingly similar symptoms are sometimes seen following cranial aneurysmal subarachnoid haemorrhage, but not as the principal feature of the condition.

Further reading

Chatterjee S, Foy PM, Findlay GF. Report of a controlled clinical trial comparing automated percutaneous lumbar discectomy and microdiscectomy in the treatment of contained lumbar disc herniation. Spine 1995; 20(6): 734–8.

Findlay GF, Hall BI, Musa BS, Oliveira MD, Fear SC. A 10-year follow-up of the outcome of lumbar microdiscectomy. Spine 1998; 23(10): 1168–71.

Freeman BJ, Fraser RD, Cain CM, Hall DJ, Chapple DC. A randomized, double-blind, controlled trial: intradiscal electrothermal therapy versus placebo for the treatment of chronic discogenic low back pain. Spine 2005; 30(21): 2369–77 (demonstrates no benefit for the technique over placebo).

Patchell RA, Tibbs PA, Regine WF, et al. Direct decompressive surgical resection in the treatment of spinal cord compression caused by metastatic cancer: a randomised trial. Lancet 2005; 366(9486): 643–8.

Porter RW, Miller CG. Neurogenic claudication and root claudication treated with calcitonin: a double blind controlled trial. Spine 1988; 13: 1061–4.

Systematic review

Gibson JNA, Wadell G, Grant JC. Surgery for degenerative lumbar spondylosis (Cochrane Review), The Cochrane Library, Issue 4, 2000. Oxford: Update Software.

Related topic of interest

Back pain – injections (p. 28); Back pain – medical management (p. 34).

BURNS

The distinction of the acute pain state from the chronic pain state is one which is discussed in other chapters in this book. Chronic pain may be considered a disease, with its own natural history and presentation and its own treatments and techniques, whereas acute pain is a simpler model and is more easily understood by a person with a conventional biomedical training. There are, however, a few areas in clinical practice where the biology and the psychology of both acute and chronic pain states must be considered simultaneously and burn injury is one such area. Observation of the way in which casualties of the Anzio invasion force of 1944 viewed their serious wounds influenced the development of the model for pain pathways that we call the 'gate control' model. On a battlefield the prospect of a safe transfer, with honour, from a place of danger to a place of safety has been said to contribute to a sense of wellbeing, even analgesia. By contrast, in civilian practice, burn casualties might be considered the most extreme example of the way in which the circumstances contribute to adverse psychological outcomes, as the gate control mechanism may not work. Burn injuries are not only physically very painful, they are associated with devastating endocrine and metabolic changes, physical changes are often permanent, and psychological consequences of, for example, facial disfigurement, or the circumstances of the incident have to be considered from the very early stages.

It is recognized too that the transition from acute to chronic pain is a process of chemical and molecular change that we call neuroplasticity. The physiological processes and chemicals involved in burn injury themselves alter the behaviour of the neurones of the dorsal horn of the spinal cord, resulting in changes in pain sensitivity. Burns have the potential for releasing most of the inflammatory mediators and mediators producing sensitization and excitation of nociceptors and intense nociceptive input that is required to produce central sensitization, a process that has been described in the laboratory setting as 'windup'. The process of dressing changes and surgery results in further trauma, and each episode of nociceptive insult to the spinal cord has the potential for provoking further changes in the behaviour of the dorsal horn neurone. The constant threat, anticipation and experience of pain, together with the modelling from examples from history, may further exacerbate the psychological distress, as well as decreasing the threshold for pain. Animal evidence on post-burn hyperalgesia, central hyperexcitability and changes in opioid sensitivity suggests that burns patients may need to be protected from developing a 'memory' of pain in neural networks.

Pain during the immediate post-burn period and during intensive management

Pain is due to the acute and ongoing pain from the burn itself and due to measures undertaken to care for the burn and prevent its complications. Full-thickness burns, even though the burnt area may be anaesthetic due to destruction of peripheral nociceptors must be considered a source of pain, as, of course, must the surrounding area where there may be less tissue damage, but intense stimulation of nociceptors. Pain in the acute period can be considered as two separate entities: a constant background pain and pain arising out of interventions such as dressings. Although strong opioid drugs are the mainstay of treatment, pain of intervention can be excruciating and inadequately controlled pharmacologically. It is accepted that there is a need for better analgesia for burn dressing changes. In this respect it is to be noted that paracetamol, nonsteroidal anti-inflammatory drugs (NSAIDs) or cyclo-oxygenase II inhibitors (COXIBs), ketamine and other NMDA anatagonists, nitrous oxide, antidepressants and anticonvulsants are often used. It is also of note that one of the largest studies of the effects of opioid safety in respect of addiction potential was undertaken on military mass burn casualties, where it was concluded that opioids used for this purpose did not lead to addiction.

Topical lidocaine 2% has been applied to skin donor sites and has been shown to reduce opioid requirements. It has also been reported as effective in partial-thickness burns, whereas intravenous lidocaine by infusion has also been reported of value. Benzodiazepines are often used as adjuncts. Lorazepam 1 mg has been reported to bring about a significant reduction in a high level of baseline pain.

Non-pharmacological interventions play an important part in the control of pain. Various cognitive, behavioural, relaxation, hypnotherapeutic and neuropsychological adjuncts have been used.

Pain persisting into the rehabilitation period

There are many mechanisms that could be reasonably expected to perpetuate the sensitized status of the dorsal horn. These include the presence of continuing low-grade noxious stimulation, the presence of nerve damage, the disordered regeneration of nerve endings into scar tissue and the presence of a degree of central nervous system sensitization at the cortical level.

The return of abnormal skin sensation is common after burn injuries and many patients complain of painful sensations and paraesthesiae in their wounds. Tactile, thermal and pain thresholds have been found to be higher in areas of burns than in non-burned patients. Deep burns injuries are more affected than superficial burns. Sensory losses were found in burned and non-burned areas, suggesting that the burned areas influence sensory perception in adjacent undamaged areas.

Patients are in the long term affected by intense itching. It is distressing and can compromise healing of newly formed fragile skin. It can occur at all stages of burn injury from 5 days to 2 years post burn, and occurs in wounds of any thickness and in donor sites. Antihistamines are used although they are not very effective. Non-pharmacological methods comprise control of ambient temperature, cool compresses, bathing, use of emollients, application of pressure, massage and the use of TENS.

Painful musculoskeletal problems may arise from deformities secondary to amputations, altered biomechanics or contractures.

Related topics of interest

Anatomy and physiology (p. 50); Neuromata, scars and chronic post-surgical pain (p. 141); Sympathetic nervous system and pain (p. 202).

CANCER PAIN – DRUGS

Cancer pain can be well or completely controlled in 80–90% of patients by following the World Health Organization (WHO) guidelines. However, 10–20% of patients will require more intensive measures to control pain. In a prospective study of 2118 patients with cancer pain managed by the WHO guidelines, 8% required nerve blocks, 3% neurolytic blocks and 3% spinal analgesia (epidural or intrathecal). Opioids are the mainstay of drug treatment in cancer pain, used either alone or in combination with other drugs. Neuropathic pain may be opioid responsive but will often require specific antineuropathic medication. Pain can also be treated by using drugs which target the pathological process responsible for the pain.

Systematic approach to drug therapy

1. Multiplicity. Most cancer patients have more than one pain; 80% have at least two pains. Pain can be caused by the tumour or its metastases, from treatments for the disease or can be unrelated to cancer, e.g. a concurrent condition.

2. Identification. Each pain must be clearly identified and treated separately.

3. Effectiveness of treatment should be regularly reviewed.

4. Efficacy. Not all pains are adequately treated by opioids. Consider the use of other opioids, antineuropathic medication or other drugs to address specifically the pathology causing pain. Doses of opioid should be increased for as long as the patient remains in pain and that pain responds to the opioid. The details of antineuropathic pain therapy is covered in other chapters.

5. Side-effects. There must be close attention to and treatment of side effects of opioid therapy.

6. Non-drug treatments might be appropriate, e.g. radiotherapy in the management of malignant bone pain. Systematic review has confirmed the benefit of radiotherapy for bone metastases. In a large study, 25% of patients had complete pain relief at 1 month and 41% had at least 50% pain relief. Radiotherapy is the treatment of choice for bone metastases.

Choice of opioid drug

Guidance to the use of analgesics in cancer pain is given by the WHO as the 'analgesic ladder'.

Step 1. If pain is mild at initial assessment, start a non-opioid such as paracetamol or a nonsteroidal anti-inflammatory drug (NSAID) regularly.

Step 2. If pain is moderate, start a weak opioid such as codeine, with a non-opioid such as paracetamol or an NSAID.

Step 3. If pain is severe, start a strong opioid such as morphine, diamorphine, hydromorphone, oxycodone with a non-opioid.

NSAIDs are recommended in metastatic bone disease or soft tissue infiltration. Recommendations are ibuprofen 200–800 mg or diclofenac 50 mg, each three tims a day by mouth.

Route of opioid

1. Oral. The oral route is preferable, unless precluded because of weakness, coma, dysphagia, vomiting or poor enteral absorption. The transdermal route can be used when there is stability in pain control. Oral opioid treatment begins at step 2 of the analgesic ladder with codeine. Codeine is a prodrug of morphine. It is available in tablets of 30 and 60 mg and in various combinations with non-opioid analgesics. Most combined analgesics contain little codeine (8–10 mg). However Tylex, Kapake and Solpadol contain 30 mg of codeine plus 500 mg of paracetamol per tablet. Recommended dose of codeine is 30–60 mg 4-hourly. Codeine is very constipating. Laxatives must be prescribed. Pain uncontrolled by codeine should be treated at step 3.

The bioavailability of morphine may be as low as 20%. It is used in two main forms: one of immediate release and one of controlled or sustained release. Immediate-release morphine is available in both liquid and tablet form. It has rapid onset, peak effect within 30–90 min, and short duration, usually of 4 hours. Modified-release morphine tablets are prescribed on a 12-hourly basis. Assessment of requirements and adjustment of dose are accomplished using the immediate-release preparation in the following way:

- Start oral morphine sulphate solution regularly (4-hourly). Dose suggested for the elderly or frail is 2.5 mg, in others 5–10 mg.
- Prescribe the same dose 2-hourly for breakthrough pain.
- If the regular dose is consistently inadequate or does not last 4 hours, increase the 4-hourly dose by 30–50%.
- Once the patient has been pain free for a period of at least 24 hour, the morphine taken in the last 24-hour period should be totalled and prescribed in controlled-release form, either as a twice-daily dose of MST (total 24-hour dose divided by two) or as a once-daily dose of the 24-hour preparations.
- One sixth of the total daily dose of morphine should always be available as oral morphine sulphate solution for breakthrough pain.
- Patients should be warned that drowsiness, dizziness and nausea may occur but wear off within a few days. Antiemetics may be necessary. Constipation is the main persistent problem, so laxatives must be prescribed.

Tramadol has a relatively low affinity for μ opioid receptors and its analgesia is only partially inhibited by naloxone, a selective μ opioid receptor antagonist. It has a second analgesic mechanism; it inhibits reuptake of serotonin and noradrenaline, thus modifying the transmission of pain impulses by enhancing serotonergic and noradrenergic pathways. The effects of the individual mechanisms in producing analgesia are modest, but in combination they are synergistic. This allows sparing of μ_2 opioid receptor side effects. Tramadol is used as a transition between weak and strong opioids. It is said to be less constipating than other opioid drugs.

Oxycodone is a strong opioid which provides an alternative to morphine if side effects of morphine are troublesome. It is 1.5–2 times as potent as oral morphine. It is available in 4-hour (immediate) and 12-hour (sustained) release preparations. Constipation can still be a problem and regular laxatives should be prescribed.

Hydromorphone is a strong opioid but has more selective μ receptor action than morphine. It is used as an alternative to morphine where side effects of morphine are troublesome. It is available in 4-hour (immediate) and 12-hour (sustained) release preparations. A conversion ratio of 7.5:1 oral morphine to oral hydromorphone is recommended, i.e. morphine 10 mg = hydromorphone 1.3 mg. Constipation can still be a problem and regular laxatives should be prescribed.

Methadone has μ and δ agonist activity. It also has some NMDA antagonist activity and so can be useful in a combined nociceptive and neuropathic pain picture. Its elimination is variable, which makes prescribing difficult.

2. Transdermal. Fentanyl is delivered transdermally in the fentanyl patch. The 25 μg h^{-1} patch is a suitable starting point with breakthrough oral morphine to allow further assessment and titration. Patches come in doses of 12, 25, 50, 75 and 100 μg h^{-1}. Each patch delivers the determined dose for 72 hours before it requires renewal. In a small number of patients the patch needs to be renewed after 48 hours. It can take 6–12 hours to achieve analgesic levels in the plasma and levels continue to rise for up to 24 hours. There is a slow fall in levels after the patch has been removed. After 17 hours plasma levels are at 50%. These kinetics must be taken into consideration in changing from one form of opioid to another. Fentanyl patches have fewer side effects than morphine, particularly constipation.

Buprenorphine may be a transdermal alternative.

3. Transmucosal. Transmucosal fentanyl can be delivered by a lozenge with applicator. It has a licence in both malignant and non-malignant pain. It is intended for breakthrough pain in those on regular strong opioids. There may be a place for it in incident pain, i.e. pain associated with movement. It is intended to be used for no more than four episodes of breakthrough pain per 24 hours. Should it be the case that satisfactory pain control is not achieved within this limit, the dose of long-acting regular opioid should be increased. The lozenge is placed against the cheek and moved around. It is kept there for 15 minutes over which time the dose within the lozenge is absorbed. It can be removed from the mouth should side effects occur during this time, and no more drug will be absorbed. This can be repeated 15 minutes later if pain control is not achieved but not again for this pain episode. Fentanyl lozenges are available in 200, 400, 600, 800, 1200 and 1600 μg doses. If two doses have been required to treat an episode of pain or if that episode has not been controlled by two doses, the next increment in lozenge size should be used at the next episode. The patient should be carefully watched during the period of dose determination.

4. Subcutaneous.   This route is used only when the oral route is not possible. Drugs are administered through a small cannula. Diamorphine is the drug of choice. (Hydromorphone is used outside Britain.) Its high solubility allows it to be dissolved in a very small volume of infusate. The potency of oral morphine to subcutaneous diamorphine is 3:1, so previous total daily oral morphine dose should be divided by three to give the 24- hour subcutaneous diamorphine dose. When infusing a volume of 10 ml per 24 hour, the subcutaneous site is effective for approximately 7 days. Breakthrough subcutaneous doses should be given at one-sixth of the 24- hour dose. The subcutaneous route is unsuitable where there is oedema, erythema, soreness, a tendency to sterile abscesses or a coagulopathy. Antiemetics and sedatives can be added to the infusate.

5. Intravenous.   This may be necessary for acute pain of malignant disease such as pathological fracture.

6. Rectal.   The oral preparations of immediate release morphine and sustained release morphine tablets can be given in suppository form.

Opioid rotation

Opioid rotation refers to a change to another opioid drug to achieve a better balance between analgesia and side effects. If the usefulness of an opioid is thought of as a continuum, side effects also determine the place of that drug on the continuum. The pharmacological principles are as follows. Tolerance is said to occur when the dose of drug needs to be increased to give the same effect. It occurs to adverse effects and to analgesic effects. Cross tolerance refers to one drug causing tolerance to another. This can apply to both analgesic and side effects. Tolerance can be less than complete. Switching to another opioid relies on cross tolerance for analgesia being less than cross tolerance for side effects. The effect of changing drug is unpredictable because equianalgesic dose cannot be predicted as it depends on the degree of cross tolerance. Some would advocate an early switch as failure to respond well to one opioid does not mean failure to respond to another.

Certain considerations must be made; there may be other causes of side effects than drug toxicity, and if pain is neuropathic it may be less responsive to opioids; consider other treatments for neuropathic pains. There are some who argue that the way to improve the side-effect–analgesia balance is to reduce the dose.

Non-narcotic analgesics

Drugs such as paracetamol, the salicylates, NSAIDs and cyclo-oxygenase type 2 inhibitors (COXIBs) are analgesics, anti-inflammatory treatments and antipyretics, with varying potencies for each of these actions.

The WHO recommends a non-narcotic analgesic for mild to moderate pain and recommends NSAIDs or COXIBs as a supplement to opioids for bone pain or soft tissue invasion. NSAIDs are of particular use when there is an inflammatory component to the pain. The use of an NSAID may allow reduction of the dosage of morphine. NSAIDs have a ceiling effect, so recommended doses should not be exceeded.

Corticosteroids

Pain with an inflammatory component can also be treated with corticosteroids. These reduce perineural oedema and are therefore used in central nervous system and spinal cord tumours. They are standard therapy for tumour-induced spinal cord compression. They are used in brachial or lumbosacral plexus invasion and can reverse early nerve compression. Pain from organ infiltration can benefit from corticosteroids. Pain from liver infiltration is improved by their effect in reducing capsular inflammation. They are given orally or intravenously. Suggested regimens are dexamethasone 2–24 mg per 24 hour orally or one-half to one-third of this dose intravenously, or prednisolone 40–100 mg per 24 hour orally. They should not be administered later than the early evening, so that sleep disturbance is avoided. Steroid enemas are used for the treatment of tenesmus.

Side effects include adrenal axis suppression, sodium and water retention and hypertension, gastritis and peptic ulceration, reduced cell-mediated immunity and increased risk of infection, mood alteration and psychoses, hyperglycaemia, increased requirements for insulin and weight gain, myopathy and osteoporosis.

Bisphosphonates

Bisphosphonates are analogues of endogenous pyrophosphates which inhibit osteoclastic bone resorption. They are claimed to be effective in the treatment of cancer-associated hypercalcaemia. Increasingly they are used to treat intractable bone pain, particularly in myeloma. Pamidronate and clodronate may be effective in reducing malignant bone pain. Clodronate can be given orally and intravenously. Pamidronate must be given by intravenous infusion. Newer bisphosphonates are zoledronate, ibandronate, aminohexane, risedronate and alendronate.

Calcitonin

Calcitonin also inhibits osteoclastic resorption of bone and is used effectively in the treatment of hypercalcaemia of malignancy. It has been said to be effective in the treatment of malignant bone pain at a dose of 100 IU twice daily subcutaneously.

Nifedipine

Nifedipine at a dose of 5–10 mg three times daily is used for the treatment of painful oesophageal spasm and the relief of tenesmus.

Hyoscine butylbromide

Colic due to malignant intestinal obstruction can be relieved by the smooth muscle relaxant hyoscine given 10–20 mg parenterally three times daily or 60–120 mg per 24 hour by subcutaneous infusion.

Oxybutinin

Painful bladder spasms may be relieved by oxybutinin. Patients should be warned of anticholinergic side effects.

Baclofen

The oral administration of baclofen, a γ-amino butyric acid (GABA) receptor agonist is used for the treatment of painful muscular spasms, 5 mg three times daily up to a maximum of 100 mg per day. It has also been used experimentally spinally. Unpleasant side effects such as sedation, fatigue and hypotonia occur.

Lidocaine

The subcutaneous infusion of lidocaine titrated against response, with attention to toxic doses, has been of effect in cancer pain.

Nitrous oxide

A mixture of 50% nitrous oxide and 50% oxygen produces analgesia without loss of consciousness. It is self-administered using a demand valve. Excessive exposure by continuous use or frequent intermittent use causes megaloblastic anaemia from interference with vitamin B_{12} synthesis. This might be considered an acceptable risk in a patient of short life expectancy.

Systematic review

McQuay HJ, Collins SL, Carroll D, Moore RA. Radiotherapy for palliation of painful bone metastases. The Cochrane Library, Issue 4, 2000. Oxford: Update Software.

CHEST PAIN

Chronic refractory angina

Chronic refractory angina is a condition which is appropriately and successfully treated in the chronic pain clinic setting. The diagnosis is made in the following circumstances:

- There is angina thought to be due to the myocardial ischaemia of advanced coronary disease despite optimal medication.
- Angioplasty or coronary artery bypass surgery have failed or are not feasible.

The diagnosis should have been agreed by cardiologist, cardiothoracic surgeon and pain clinician. There should be regular cardiological review to ensure the patient has not developed new disease that needs revascularization and for supervision of antianginal medication. Assessment should ensure that the patient has in fact failed to respond and that poor compliance is not the cause. Similarly, obvious alternative diagnoses such as pain resulting from hyperacidity syndromes of the upper gastrointestinal tract need excluding before further management of the chest pain is contemplated: a trial of proton pump inhibitor should be considered. Pharmacological treatment should be rationalized in a multidisciplinary setting. A psychosocial history will help identify stressors and inappropriate beliefs, as well as helping to identify depression and anxiety.

Epidemiology

Chronic refractory angina consumes a large amount of resources. A typical patient referred to a chronic refractory angina clinic has a severely curtailed quality of life and is demanding of medical resources. The average patient with chronic refractory angina uses resources, per annum, as follows:

- General practitioner surgery visits: 6.5
- Hospital outpatient visits: 3.59
- Hospital admissions: 1.72
- GP home visits: 1.44
- Hospital emergency visits: 0.55

Symptom scoring is as follows:

- Mean pain severity score = 6.6
- Mean limitation of activity = 58%

Co-morbidity

Incidence of other symptoms is as follows:

- Anxiety = 79.4%
- Depression = 58%

In addition it will be recognized that these patients have been failed by the traditional model of disease that has taught them and their carers that angina is a sign of imminent catastrophe! The pain clinician will appreciate that it is possible to change the way in which such fear is addressed. Angina that is refractory to medical treatment can be considered as a pain syndrome with much in common with other visceral pain syndromes. The authors of the National Refractory Angina Guideline make the following suggestions for management, recognizing that individual patients vary in their responsiveness for particular treatments. The Guideline recommends a stepwise approach, in order of increasing invasiveness, risk of complications and cost. Where effect and duration have been favourable, there is a case to repeat treatments and possibly provide them on a regular basis as need arises, e.g. temporary sympathetic blockade. The Guideline recommends:

Counselling
Explanation of the management plan and lifestyle advice.

Rehabilitation
Rehabilitation may reduce mortality and has been shown to reduce morbidity and symptom reporting and improve quality of life. Relaxation and stress management have both been shown to reduce angina.

Multidisciplinary cognitive behavioural pain management programme
The most effective rehabilitation intervention has been shown to be exercise combined with psychological input.

Transcutaneous electrical nerve stimulation
The mechanism of TENS in angina is unknown. It is used at continuous high frequency (70 Hz) for 1 hour three times a day and during angina attacks. Stronger stimulation may be needed during attacks. If it is to be used in a patient with a pacemaker, the pacemaker may require reprogramming. The TENS machine should be trialled in the safety of the pacemaker clinic. The effect of TENS during an acute attack is usually immediate.

Temporary sympathetic blockade
Angina involves the activation of afferent sympathetic pathways. Temporary interruption of sympathetic innervation can have an effect on pain. The effect and its duration are however not predictable.

In two-thirds of patients sympathetic relay is at the level of the stellate ganglion and in one-third it is at a low thoracic level. It was recognized as early as 1930 that infiltration of the stellate ganglion with local anaesthetic relieved angina and this has been substantiated by further studies. The injection of 15 ml of 0.5% bupivacaine to the left stellate ganglion can give lasting relief. Logically therefore, the stellate ganglion is the first choice for blockade, but the thoracic chain can be considered as a (more invasive) option in cases of failure to respond. Thoracic sympathetic blockade is performed by the injection of 15 ml of 0.5% bupivacaine at the paravertebral T3/4 level on the left side or by thoracic epidural at the same level. High thoracic epidural may achieve the same.

Spinal cord stimulation

Spinal cord stimulation (SCS) is used for prophylaxis or for the treatment of acute attacks. It has been shown to improve symptoms, quality of life, reduce number of ischaemic episodes, reduce glyceryl trinitrate consumption and reduce number of hospital admissions. It makes myocardial blood flow more homogenous, thereby redistributing flow to areas which were previously ischaemic. An electrode is placed epidurally in the C7/T2 region under X-ray control. The level is adjusted to induce paraesthesia in the areas affected by the angina. It does not mask the pain of myocardial infarction and there is no increase in mortality rates in those who have a stimulator compared with those who do not. Chronic refractory angina responds well to SCS.

Opioids

Opioids may be effective in relieving refractory angina. A careful trial is recommended. There may be a place for the intrathecal infusion of opioids.

Interventional cardiology/minimally invasive techniques

Destructive sympathectomy and laser myocardial revascularization are procedures which may be tried in some centres.

Non-cardiac chest pain

A substantial proportion of patients referred to cardiologists do not have underlying coronary artery disease, but are disabled by symptoms identical to angina. The condition cryptically referred to as syndrome X represents a group of such patients who demonstrate abnormalities of ECG on exercise testing but have normal coronary arteries on angiography. In such patients the cause of the pain has been variously described as due to microvascular occlusion, or due to alteration of the way in which the endothelial lining of blood vessels responds to local constrictor and dilator substances. These patients are amenable to the management strategies outlined above, with the added opportunity to address the symptoms as they would be in any other condition where the pain is not indicative of a life-threatening condition. As expected, the patient with non-cardiac chest pain or syndrome X presents with symptoms of psychological distress. A link between anxiety disorders and non-cardiac chest pain has been demonstrated, as has the high prevalence of panic disorder and depressive illness.

Management

The same principles apply as to the management of refractory angina. Here, however, there is no potential life-threatening condition to which the symptoms may be attributed. Imipramine and clonidine have been shown to reduce the frequency of episodes of chest pain, whereas sertraline reduces pain intensity. Cognitive behavioural therapy, particularly that which addresses the issues of catastrophizing and coping strategies, has been shown to be effective.

Other chest pains

Pathology of the lungs and its associated structures can cause chronic pain. The pleuritic pain of interpleural adhesions from acute inflammatory disease can be treated with physiotherapy and nonsteroidal anti-inflammatory drugs (NSAIDs).

An estimated 65% of adult cystic fibrosis presents with chest pain, the majority of these being in the last 6 months of life. The history usually reveals a worsening of pain over a 2-year period. The pain is severe and usually in the anterior inferior part of the chest but may flit. It is exacerbated by coughing and breathing. It is a dull aching sensation felt to be within the tissue of the lungs and not in the chest wall. Whether it is a pre-terminal event or whether it seriously impedes expectoration and therefore precipitates death is unclear but the weight of opinion favours the latter. As such, this is a serious problem which kills. Formal quantitative sensory testing at one of the UK's leading neuropathic pain research centres has found the pain to be nociceptive.

It has been found to be unresponsive to paracetamol, ibuprofen and carbamazepine.

Opioids may have an adverse effect on pulmonary function and the constipation they cause results in problems in patients who require pancreatic supplementation for their malabsorption.

There are reports of the treatment of the pain by continuous epidural infusion but this is not without potential complications in this group of patients at risk of serious infections with atypical organisms. Capsaicin cream has been found to be partially effective in some patients but loses its usefulness as it causes an irritating cough in this group.

A pain similar in characteristic is seen in other chronic lung disease sufferers.

Further reading

National Refractory Angina Guidelines: www.angina.org

COMPLEX REGIONAL PAIN SYNDROMES

The complex regional pain syndromes (CRPS) comprise a variety of clinical presentations in which severe pain is associated with vasomotor changes and dysfunction in response to injury. Previously known as reflex sympathetic dystrophy and causalgia, the latter being a description of the presentation following specific nerve injury, they were reclassified in 1994 in an attempt to distance the syndromes from the implication that the sympathetic nervous system was always involved in the pathophysiology. However, the new taxonomy is by no means universally accepted, and references to the old taxonomy are regularly found in the literature. The syndromes also include conditions known as 'shoulder–hand syndrome', 'Sudeck's atrophy' and 'algodystrophy.' The complex regional pain syndromes are neuropathic pain syndromes (type 2 is defined by the presence of nerve injury as the primary mechanism).

Definitions and diagnostic criteria

Complex regional pain syndrome type 1

Complex regional pain syndrome type 1 may follow an injury or event that causes immobilization. There are three mandatory criteria for diagnosis:

1. Continuing pain, allodynia (painful response to normally non-noxious stimulus) or hyperalgesia (heightened response to a painful stimulus) for which the pain is disproportionate to any inciting event.
2. Evidence at some time of oedema, changes in skin blood flow or abnormal sudomotor (sweating) activity in the region of pain.
3. Diagnosis is excluded by presence of conditions which would otherwise account for the pain and dysfunction.

Complex regional pain syndrome type 2

1. Continuing pain, allodynia or hyperalgesia following a nerve injury, not necessarily limited to the distribution of the nerve.
2. Evidence at some time of oedema, changes in skin blood flow or abnormal sudomotor activity in the region of pain.
3. Diagnosis is excluded by presence of conditions which would otherwise account for the pain and dysfunction.

There is a good deal of heterogeneity in the presenting symptoms, but allodynia with draughts and clothing and extreme sensitivity to temperature changes are common. Type 2 often presents with allodynia combined with hypoaesthesia. Although the above criteria are sensitive, they are not specific, and a further diagnostic criterion is thus proposed.

Complex regional pain syndrome consists of pain that is disproportionate to any inciting event, and includes reports of at least one symptom in each of the following three categories:

- Sensory: reports of hyperaesthesia.
- Vasomotor: reports of temperature and/or skin colour change and/or skin colour asymmetry.
- Motor/trophic: reports of decreased range of motion and/or motor dysfunction (weakness, tremor or dystonia) and/or trophic changes (hair, nail, skin).

Signs are reported in two or more of the following categories:

- Sensory: evidence of hyperalgesia to pin prick and/or allodynia.
- Vasomotor: evidence of temperature asymmetry and/or skin colour changes and/or asymmetry.
- Sudomotor/oedema: evidence of any of these and/or asymmetry.
- Motor/trophic: evidence of impairment, dysfunction or trophic change

The presentation may be complicated by a 'half body' sensory impairment and motor neglect of the affected limb. In addition, the affected limb may 'feel foreign', a phenomenon known as 'cognitive neglect'. The temperature changes are commonly described as an initial 'warm phase' followed by a 'cold phase'. This is believed to be due to alterations in cutaneous sympathetic vasoconstrictor activity but may also reflect changes in central sensory processing.

The diagnosis of CRPS remains a clinical one, and the role of such investigations as have been suggested is controversial. Clinical tests to establish the degree of impairment of the sensory and vasomotor systems include quantitative sensory testing, thermographic imaging and laser Doppler fluxmetry. These may be used to follow the progress of the condition and its response to treatment.

Pathophysiology

This is unknown. There are several theories.

1. Autonomic nervous system. Classically the inappropriate reaction of the sympathetic nervous system was implicated. This is a view that has been challenged. Autonomic involvement is often a feature but is inconstant and varies with time. Abnormalities of blood flow are demonstrated. This may be attributed to the sympathetic nervous system causing reflex vasomotor spasm and subsequent loss of vascular tone. However, gross limb blood flow is also related to the degree of muscle inactivity. It is thought that increased blood flow may cause excessive bone resorption to account for secondary osteoporotic changes. The degree of osteoporosis is often disproportionate to the degree of disuse. Neither definition (type 1 nor 2) requires the role of the sympathetic nervous system in the maintenance of the symptoms, although it is tempting to assume that symptoms of temperature change, skin blood flow and alterations in sweating are being mediated by the sympathetic nervous system. Blockade of the sympathetic system to the affected part has variable effects, and this may make for secondary differential diagnoses of 'sympathetically mediated' (SMP) and 'sympathetic independent' (SIP) pain.

2. Inflammation. CRPS has signs in common with acute inflammatory processes, namely changes in colour and temperature and the presence of swelling and pain. There is experimental evidence of disturbance of mitochondrial oxygenation. Oxygen extraction in the affected region has been shown to be impaired. Free radicals may be involved in this inflammatory reaction. However, the innate cytokine profile in patients with complex regional pain syndrome is normal. An autoimmune aetiology has also been suggested.

3. Inactivity. Immobilization or reluctance to use the affected limb severely exacerbates the syndrome and results in secondary changes such as localized osteoporosis, muscle contractures and muscle atrophy. Immobility reduces blood circulation: poor flow may account for the trophic changes seen in skin and nails. Rat models show that immobilization alone can generate a syndrome resembling CRPS, with substance P signalling contributing to the vascular and nociceptive changes observed.

4. Central pain. Although no clear mechanism has been defined, nor any clear link demonstrated, the development of CRPS after traumatic spinal cord injury and the presence of a similar syndrome in stroke victims suggest there could be a central mechanism.

5. Psychological factors. CRPS is a chronic condition and, as expected, the patient's beliefs and prior experience of illness and injury will have bearing on the potential for recovery. Stressful life events are more common in patients with CRPS, but the stressful life events are risk factors and not causes of CRPS.

6. A complex disease of the peripheral and central nervous system. Abnormal integration of the somatosensory, sympathetic and somatomotor systems takes place at several levels, with the end result being an abnormal response of neural nociceptive tissue causing 'neurogenic inflammation' at the periphery. According to this theory, the initial insult occurs in the periphery and triggers changes in the central representation of the sensory, motor and sympathetic systems, which are reflected in the changes of the respective output systems observed in CRPS patients. Subsequent interactions with the immune, endocrine and vascular systems leads to changes in the long-term responsiveness of the central nervous system. The description of physiological changes without pain, the so-called complex regional painless syndrome, further supports the idea of a self-sustaining abnormal physiological response to an initial assault. Even more supportive of the idea of a complex disease affecting the central nervous system is the observed association between CRPS and dystonia.

Experimental basis for the complexity of peripheral and central processing abnormalities. Various techniques support the concept that CRPS is a physiological disturbance of the central and peripheral nervous system:

- Impairment of sympathetic vasoconstriction in a limb affected by CRPS is observed after central vasoconstrictor stimulation is applied.
- A technique in which protein extravasation from tissue after electrical stimulation through microelectrodes can be observed shows that patients

with CRPS respond in a manner similar to volunteers pretreated with the inflammatory mediator substance P.

- In-vivo proton magnetic resonance spectroscopy has also suggested that central neuronal chemistry is altered in patients with CRPS and there is also evidence of central reorganization.
- Functional MRI scanning has demonstrated particular changes in brain processing during mechanical hyperalgesia in CRPS.

Epidemiology

Lack of uniform terminology and diagnostic criteria has hitherto confounded attempts to determine the incidence of CRPS. CRPS type 1 has been described in children, but the incidence is much lower than in adults. CRPS may occur in 1–2% of patients after fractures and in 2–5% of patients after peripheral nerve injury. There is no correlation between severity of initial injury and likelihood of developing CRPS; indeed, in some series, no precipitating cause can be ascertained in 10–26% of cases. Some series have reported a higher incidence in the Caucasian population. Genetic studies have suggested that the HLA types A3, B7 and DR2 confer a risk, with the DR2 type associated with a poorer response to treatment. However, these racial and genetic differences may be more a result of patient selection bias than a true finding.

Prognosis

There are conflicting reports regarding prognosis. One study claimed as many as 80% of patients with initial symptoms of CRPS type 1 were 'cured' within 18 months from onset, spontaneously or with treatment. By contrast, another study of CRPS, consisting of 1348 patients, reported that 96% of the study subjects still suffered some pain and disability regardless of the duration of the disease or course of treatment. Greater duration of CRPS is related to significantly greater likelihood of abnormalities of sensation and less likelihood of sweating abnormalities or oedema. Most children with CRPS show reduced pain and improved function with a non-invasive rehabilitative treatment approach. Long-term functional outcomes were also very good.

Management

There are many theories as to how to treat CRPS but the ideal progression through various treatment modalities has not been established. Management involves reducing the disability as well as the pain and the distress. Persuading the patient to move the affected limb is an important part of management. Attempts to modify the sympathetic nervous system are commonly used in an attempt to provide analgesia. There are three strategies that have to be considered: intravenous sympathetic block, sympathetic ganglion block and the use of drugs acting on the nervous system. There are, however, a paucity of randomized controlled studies to justify the use of these treatments.

1. Intravenous sympathetic block using guanethidine in a limb isolated by a tourniquet is a commonly performed procedure, is easy to perform and is often repeated. The evidence for its effectiveness, as assessed by randomized controlled trials, however, is far from convincing. A strong placebo effect has been noted, and it is possible that the analgesic effect claimed is a consequence of ischaemia and pressure on the peripheral nerves from the tourniquet leading to an alteration of function during the recovery period. Guanethidine is a drug with important cardiovascular side effects if released into the systemic circulation (after, for example, premature deflation of the tourniquet). Thus there is a degree of controversy over the continued place of this procedure. In addition to guanethidine, various claims have been made for a variety of drugs, including bretylium, clonidine, ketanserin and reserpine, to be used in an isolated tourniquet technique. Local anaesthetic is usually injected with guanethidine to provide immediate pain relief and to prevent the pain of injection of the supposedly active drug. This will give a degree of analgesia that outlasts the tourniquet application and may allow a 'window of opportunity' for the patient to regain the ability to move the affected limb. Hence it is difficult to separate any claimed 'general' benefit of the procedure from the 'specific' benefit of the drug.

2. Sympathetic ganglion block is another frequently used procedure for CRPS of the limbs. Stellate ganglion block is used to block the sympathetic outflow of the upper thoracic ganglia that provide sympathetic fibres to the upper limb, and lumbar sympathetic block of the lumbar ganglia for the lower limb. The use of the latter has historically been associated with the use of open surgical techniques to destroy the lumbar sympathetic chain. More recently, thoracoscopic techniques have allowed the same procedure to be undertaken on the thoracic chain, and percutaneous chemical and radiofrequency lesioning techniques on the lumbar chain.

Tempting as it is to treat the patient who responds to a local anaesthetic block with a neurodestructive one, the long-term results are unconvincing. There are significant risks: neuritis of the genitofemoral nerve in the case of chemical lumbar sympathectomy occurs despite accuracy in placing the needle on the sympathetic chain. The long-term effects of denervation of the sympathetic efferent system on the postsynaptic receptor population cannot be ignored: there is a risk of stimulation of sensitive postsynaptic receptors by circulating catecholamines. In addition a 'permanently' vasodilated and warm limb may be at best an inconvenience, at worst a source of distress.

It is suggested that the very variable responses to sympathetic nerve destruction are the consequences of the very varied types of presentation and pathophysiology in CRPS. It is further suggested that progress in the future will depend on a reliable 'diagnostic test' for the involvement of the sympathetic nervous system in individual cases, allowing the clinician to avoid a potentially futile procedure if the pain is not relieved by the diagnostic test. To this end the intravenous phentolamine test was proposed. This requires the intravenous administration of phentolamine by infusion. In practice, however, phentolamine testing requires the admission to hospital for a technique that involves cardiovascular risks similar to those of guanethidine intravenous block.

In summary, local anaesthetic blocks of the sympathetic nervous system may in some cases deliver short- to intermediate-term pain relief, but the ability to predict long-term success with nerve destruction is unproven. The management of CRPS requires measures over and above an attempt to provide analgesia. It is vitally important that the patient is encouraged to regain normal function. This can be achieved under cover of repeated local anaesthetic blocks or local anaesthetic infusion of a nerve plexus without recourse to an attempt to provide a 'permanent' solution.

The difficulty with assessing the effective treatments for CRPS lies with the varied presentations, the differing requirements of patients and the different expectations of patients and clinicians. For example, a clinical trial that has as its criterion for success a 50% reduction in pain severity may fail to recognize as a positive effect a very substantial reduction of disability or a lesser degree of pain relief that enables the patient to sleep or function properly. The continuing enthusiasm for sympathetic blocks by clinicians and patients despite poor 'high level' evidence may reflect the experience gained by many over many years.

3. Drug management. The action of certain antidepressants and anticonvulsants in neuropathic pain has been established, and so their use in CRPS, which by definition involves neuropathic pain mechanisms, is justified. However, as with sympathetic block, it is important not to lose sight of the purpose of treatment, which is to persuade the patient to continue to move the limb, and in practice, any strategy which enables this to happen is acceptable.

Other interventions

Other interventions, medications, injection techniques and cognitive behavioural therapy may be introduced when the patient appears to be failing to make progress through the steps in the pathway. Some of these techniques have been investigated with controlled trials: there is evidence to support the use of spinal cord stimulation. Sham acupuncture does not differ from acupuncture in its effect. Case reports in the literature suggest that intrathecal bupivacaine helps symptoms but does not affect the natural outcome of CRPS type 1. As might be expected for a diverse collection of symptoms that represent the CRPS, many therapies have been advocated. They include:

Drugs
- Bisphosphonates.
- Nifedipine.
- DMSO.
- *N*-acetyl cysteine.
- Subcutaneous lidocaine.
- Ketamine infusion.
- Topical capsaicin.
- Intrathecal baclofen.

Other techniques
- Electroconvulsive therapy.
- Transcranial magnetic stimulation.
- Hyperbaric oxygen.
- Mirror visual feedback therapy.

- Peripheral nerve stimulation.

The various treatment options can be justified in terms of the particular targets on which they are believed to work and which may be contributing to the symptom complex at peripheral and central level.

Potential peripheral pathophysiological targets (and possible treatments)
- Abnormal responsiveness of peripheral afferent fibers mediated by inflammatory and other algogenic substances:
    somatosensory blocks, corticosteroids.
- Altered levels of expression and functioning of multiple ion channels:
    local anaesthetics, calcium channel blockers, anticonvulsants.
- Abnormal interneuronal communication, and increased peripheral expression of adrenergic receptors and sympathetic excitation:
    sympathetic blocks, α-adrenergic antagonists, α$_2$ agonists.

Central pathophysiological targets (and possible treatments)
- Reorientation of dorsal horn terminals:
    desensitization techniques.
- Functional reduction in inhibitory interneurone activity:
    tricyclic antidepressants, gabapentin, opioids.
- Central sensitization and increased central excitability:
    gabapentin, topiramate, spinal cord stimulation, somatosensory blocks.
- Impaired descending nociceptive inhibition:
    tricyclic antidepressants, opioids.
- Adaptive changes in the cortical centres underlying the sensory-discriminative and affective-motivational dimensions of pain:
    psychological, physical and occupational therapies.

The treatment choices should be aimed at remodulating, normalizing, disrupting or preventing the progression of abnormalities in pain processing. Local anaesthetic sympathetic nerve blocks routinely performed will assess the contribution of the sympathetic nervous system. To the extent that peripheral somatosensory nerve blocks can diminish nociceptive input to the central nervous system, these techniques may help reduce the nociceptive sensitization of spinal neurones. Pain relief, however it is achieved and however temporary it is, is intended to facilitate participation in functional therapies to normalize use and to improve motion, strength and dexterity. Psychological therapies, such as biofeedback and cognitive behavioural techniques targeting pain, stress and mood disorders, are valuable adjunctive treatments for pain control and can facilitate functional improvement. The use of a mirror placed so as to give the patient a view of the reflection of the contralateral limb instead of the affected one is an example of a technique used to promote positive imagery that can be used to encourage exercise and activity of an affected limb. The effectiveness of this technique demonstrates the complex central mechanisms involved in modulating the pain and loss of function. The management of CRPS is a rehabilitation exercise, involving a stepwise progression through various physical and occupational therapy strategies.

Rehabilitation

The steps in rehabilitation are as follows:

- Reactivation.
- Densitization.

Progressing to:

- Flexibility.
- Oedema control.
- Peripheral electrical stimulation.
- Isometric strengthening.
- Treatment of secondary myofascial pain.

Progressing to:

- Gentle increase in range of motion.
- Stress loading.
- Isotonic strengthening.
- Gentle aerobic conditioning.
- Postural normalization.

Progressing to:

- Ergonomics.
- Movement therapies.
- Normalization of use.
- Vocational and functional rehabilitation.

Oedema is managed by bandaging and lymph flow massage. Movement is optimized by scrubbing (for the upper limb, literally becoming able to scrub a floor on all fours with progressive force onto the scrubbing brush, or for the lower limb attaching the scrubbing brush to the foot) and other physiotherapy modalities such as extending range of movement, activity increase, strengthening and flexibility. Gait and posture correction and treatment of associated myofascial pains, e.g. in the proximal joint, are also carried out by the physiotherapist.

Prevention

One case series suggests benefit from the use of prophylactic stellate ganglion block in patients with CRPS type 1 who are undergoing surgery on the affected upper extremity. The finding of an impaired sympathetic vasoconstrictor response when testing the vasoconstrictor response to sympathetic stimuli – recorded with laser Doppler fluxmetry – in patients who go on to develop CRPS type 1 suggests that this may serve as a marker that might be useful to intensify early therapy on patients where it might be most effective.

Conclusion

Complex regional pain syndrome is a heterogeneous disorder that falls in the spectrum of neuropathic pain disorders. It is maintained by abnormalities throughout the neuraxis (the peripheral, autonomic and central nervous systems). The pathophysiology of CRPS is not fully known. There are no scientifically well-established treatments. The diagnostic criteria for CRPS at this time are purely clinical, and the use of diagnostic tests has not been validated.

Management of CRPS uses a multidisciplinary approach, with the inclusion of medical and psychological intervention, and physical and occupational therapy. The key is gradual, persistent, functional improvement. The rational use of pain therapies must be grounded in a thorough knowledge of the neurobiology of pain, its endogenous modulation and the clinical presentation.

Further reading

Baron R, Fields HL, Janig W, Kitt C, Levine JD. National Institutes of Health Workshop: reflex sympathetic dystrophy/complex regional pain syndromes – state-of-the-science. Anesthesia and Analgesia 2002; 95: 1812–16.

Harden RN. A clinical approach to complex regional pain syndrome. The Clinical Journal of Pain 2000; 16(2): 26–32.

Jang W, Stanton-Hicks M, eds. Reflex Sympathetic Dystrophy: A Re-appraisal. Seattle: IASP Press, 1989.

Kingery WS. A critical review of controlled clinical trials for peripheral neuropathic pain and complex regional pain syndromes, Pain 1997; 73(2): 123–39.

Paice E. Fortnightly review: reflex sympathetic dystrophy. British Medical Journal 1995; 310: 1645–7.

Schott GD. Interrupting the sympathetic outflow in causalgia and reflex sympathetic dystrophy: a futile procedure for many patients. British Medical Journal 1998; 316: 792–3.

Stanton-Hicks M, Burton AW, Bruehl SP, et al. An updated interdisciplinary clinical pathway for CRPS: report of an expert panel. Pain Practice 2002; 2: 1–6.

Systematic review

Jadad AR, Carroll D, Glynn CJ, McQuay HJ. Intravenous regional sympathetic blockade for pain relief in reflex sympathetic dystrophy: a systematic review and a randomised double-blind crossover study. Journal of Pain and Symptom Management 1995; 10: 13–20.

Related topics of interest

Anatomy and physiology (p. 5); Nerve blocks – sympathetic system (p. 124); Sympathetic nervous system and pain (p. 202).

DEPRESSION AND PAIN

Pain and depression may occur concomitantly. Chronic pain may exacerbate depression. Chronic pain may be exacerbated by depression. The relative contribution and effect of each illness can be difficult to determine. Patients may not appreciate being questioned about symptoms of depression when they are consulting about symptoms of pain, but it is valuable to obtain a relevant history of symptoms of depression as a consequence of pain. In practice there is a risk that asking specific questions about depression may lead to a patient drawing a conclusion that the clinician is not taking the symptom of pain seriously. There is also a risk that important symptoms may be missed by the pain clinician. A multidisciplinary approach to patients who appear to be depressed may be of value. Conversely, expert opinion from a pain clinician about effective therapy may be valuable for the psychiatrist who otherwise may be tempted to explain the pain symptoms in terms of a depressive illness. There is a third reason for close liaison. This is that while antidepressant drugs are useful analgesics in a number of painful conditions, the most effective of these (tricyclics) have side effects and are dangerous in cases of an overdose. In general terms, a clear diagnosis of depression requires proper and safe management of depression, even if this means antidepressant drugs which have limited analgesic effectiveness. An attempt to treat pain and depression simultaneously with one drug such as a tricyclic antidepressant may be possible, but the risk of overdose should be assessed and managed before this is done.

Chronic pain exacerbating depression

An estimated 28% of patients attending pain clinics have a well-defined affective illness. A greater number are dysphoric. Factors which worsen mood in a patient suffering from chronic pain are the inability to work, the futility of medical intervention and suggestions of their malingering. Patients become depressed during the course of a painful illness when they have not been depressed previously.

Chronic pain exacerbated by depression

Approximately half of all depressed patients have pain. Atypical facial pain was the most common presenting symptom in 66% of a series of depressed women. In a smaller proportion of both sexes, tension headache was the most common presenting symptom of depression. Sites of pains which can be symptoms of depression are, in order of frequency, face, head, low back, limbs and abdomen. Characteristics of patients in whom pain may be a symptom of depression are low self-esteem, disturbed family circumstances, a personal history of psychological problems or a family history of psychiatric illness.

Assessment of depressive symptoms in the chronic pain clinic

The additional presence of biological symptoms of depression such as loss of appetite and sleeplessness indicates that pain might be a symptom of depression. Self-rating questionnaires such as the Beck depression inventory, the Zung depression scale and the Hospital Anxiety and Depression scale are used. These tests do not constitute a full assessment, nor a psychiatric diagnostic process. They are quick, simple screening tools, alerting the interviewer to a possible problem that may need further detailed questioning.

The need to distinguish depression from chronic pain

Unfortunately the common use of antidepressants and the presence of common features results in a blurring of distinctions in which it might be thought irrelevant to make an effort to diagnose depression in chronic pain patients. The distinction is important, however, if only because the doses of tricyclic antidepressant required for treatment of each condition are very different. Analgesic effect is independent of antidepressant effect. This is supported by evidence of an analgesic effect in euthymic patients, by the early response of chronic pain to amitriptyline compared with the later response of depression and by the effectiveness of amitriptyline in the treatment of chronic pain at doses much lower than those required to treat depression. An important principle of chronic pain management is that pain may be an illness in itself and not a symptom of other disease. This concept is untenable if other diseases, including depression, can account for the symptoms. Small doses of antidepressants, as used for pain management, may not be adequate. The use of invasive pain management techniques in a patient who is primarily depressed risks failure as well as the inherent risks of the procedure. Formal assessment of mental state protects against futile or potentially damaging medical intervention.

Management of depressive symptoms in the chronic pain clinic

Support for the pain clinic may be provided by clinical psychologists or liaison psychiatrists. Psychologists are able to offer cognitive and behavioural treatments for depression in which negative thoughts and beliefs can be challenged and strategies developed for improving mood and psychological well-being. Cognitive treatment may be ineffective if mood is very low, or severe biological symptoms are present, in which case medical management of depression is necessary.

Common mechanisms for pain and depression

A group of euthymic patients with pain without a physical explanation was found to have an increased family history of depressive disorders. The pain responded to the use of antidepressants. Although at present distinctions are made in diagnosis and treatment, the interaction between pain and depression and the effectiveness of antidepressants in both illnesses suggests involvement of noradrenaline and serotonin in both. The role of common neurotransmitters suggests common pathology. This fact may be valuable when offering an explanation to the patient who is sceptical of the interest in depressive symptoms that the pain clinician is taking.

Psychiatric nomenclature and chronic pain

The science of nomenclature of mental health problems allows experts from all professions in mental health to define syndromes using common diagnostic criteria. Some of these classifications have been used to describe conditions in which pain is experienced. The Diagnostic and Statistical Manual (DSM) classification of the American Psychiatric Association is one such system. The fourth version of this system (known as DSM IV) recognizes a condition called 'pain disorder', or what is in this book referred to as 'the chronic pain syndrome', as a specific syndrome. Pain disorder, according to this classification, is diagnosed when the following preconditions are met:

- Pain is the predominant presenting complaint.
- Pain causes significant distress or impairment in social, occupational or other important areas of functioning.
- Psychological factors are considered to play a significant role in the onset, severity, exacerbation or maintenance of the pain.
- The patient is not malingering.
- There is no better explanation, i.e. a mood, anxiety or depressive disorder.

DSM IV represents an advance on its predecessor, DSM III. DSM III described a condition called 'psychogenic pain'. This was defined as 'pain as an expression of psychopathology'. Although this recognized the importance of psychological factors in the pain experience, it implied an unhelpful dichotomy between physical and psychological causes, leading to an assumption that pain was either physical or 'in the mind'. This dichotomy is, unfortunately, too often reinforced when conventional medical thinking attempts to tackle a patient with the chronic pain syndrome, or the clinician cannot explain the symptoms and is looking for a 'way out' to refer the patient on to psychology services.

The WHO International Classification of Diseases (ICD) version 10 is a parallel system to the DSM taxonomy. ICD refers to 'persistent somatoform pain disorder' as persistent distressing severe pain which cannot be fully explained by a physical disorder or physiological process, and 'somatization disorder', a condition associated with a poor prognosis and in which pain is one of many symptoms, such as breathlessness and abdominal bloating present over many years. Both diagnoses assume psychosocial causative factors.

The DSM IV taxonomy has taken the terms 'somatization disorder' and 'psychological factors affecting pain' out of the nomenclature in the belief that such classifications, as variants on the more comprehensive description 'pain disorder' suffer from the same disadvantages as the term psychogenic pain.

There are obvious advantages in the recognition of the condition called 'pain disorder' or 'chronic pain syndrome' into a mental health classification system. Significant amongst these is the realization that psychological factors may need to be addressed, with a chance for improvement. Responsibility for the management of the condition by professionals with a backgound in mental health problems is also recognized. For practical purposes we would recommend that the clinician who is not a specialist in mental health disorders satisfies himself or herself with the more comprehensive description of 'pain syndrome', rather than trying to justify the term 'somatization' to colleagues or patients.

Further reading

APA DSM IV TR Text: American Psychiatric Association, Washington, DC, 2000.

Related topics of interest

Psychosocial assessment (p. 181); Therapy – antidepressants (p. 209).

FACIAL PAIN

There are many causes and clinical syndromes of facial pain. This is attributed to one or more of the following reasons:

- There are many anatomical structures in close proximity.
- There is significant representation of facial sensation within the cerebral cortex.
- The face plays a vital role in personal and social interaction.

The syndromes also cross-over into the realm of headache; and the patient may present to any one of a number of specialities: pain clinicians, maxillofacial surgeons, ENT surgeons, neurologists and neurosurgeons, each of whom may specialize in the treatment of one or more of the diagnoses. It follows that a correct diagnosis is essential, so a section of this chapter is devoted to the principles of differential diagnosis in this situation, which is often difficult. The importance of psychosocial factors should not be underestimated: what the patient thinks about the significance of the pain has an important bearing on its perception, the degree of impairment and the way it is treated.

Temporomandibular joint disorders

Temporomandibular joint disease

This is taken to mean pain arising from the temporomandibular joint (TMJ) and the masticatory muscles. Temporomandibular joint disease occurs in a milder form equally in both sexes but those presenting for treatment (approximately 5–10% of the population) are female in a ratio of 8:1.

TMJ disease is best understood by considering it to be two separate pathologies: first, temporomandibular joint dysfunction (TMJD), considered primarily to be a myofascial disorder; secondly, a true disorder of the joint itself, referred to here as 'internal derangement of the TMJ' – historically the eponym 'Costen's syndrome' has been applied to these disorders, though in a rather non-specific manner. In the first instance the reader is referred also to the sections on myofascial pain syndromes. Although it is appropriate to treat TMJD in the pain clinic, true disorders of the TMJ are the province of maxillo-facial surgeons. Their expertise is often required initially to distinguish these two conditions.

Temporomandibular joint dysfunction

The validity of various aetiological theories such as occlusal derangement and bruxism remains unknown. Temporomandibular pain may be another form of musculoskeletal pain syndrome, and the sufferer may experience the same psychological consequences as the sufferer from one of these syndromes. The similarity between non-specific low back pain and temporomandibular pain has been mentioned by some authorities. The futility, and indeed danger, of adopting a purely biomedical view of the problem is the same – it leads to over-investigation and unnecessary invasive treatment. These treatments have included prosthetic implants into the temporomandibular joint which have subsequently shown to be harmful.

Presentation. There is intermittent pain of the ear, angle of the mandible or temple or it can be less well localized. It can be bilateral. It is more intense in the morning or afternoon. It is exacerbated by movement or clenching. It may be associated with joint noises and reduced range of joint movement. There is tenderness of the joint capsule and muscles of mastication and trigger points can often be elicited. It lasts from weeks to years. Classically the pain is altered by the palpation of associated tender muscles and alleviated by the stretching of the muscle or the injection of local anaesthetic to the tender site.

Treatment. Where the myofascial dysfunction is secondary to an occlusal problem, treatment of the underlying cause may benefit. The correction of occlusal abnormality resulting from an orthodontic problem or improperly filled tooth is necessary. Splinting devices are commonly used to this end. The difficulties in proving the benefit of such appliances are considerable. By 1995, 26 randomized controlled trials of 15 different splint devices had been identified. In the systematic review in which this was reported, a high placebo response rate was noted. A second systematic review reported a benefit of splint therapy in three controlled trials out of 14. As far as other symptoms are concerned, it is of interest that an occlusal splint was more effective for prevention of migraine than a placebo intraoral device which did not alter occlusion.

In addition to the management of occlusal problems, the following approaches have been reported of use in the treatment of muscle spasm. Injections to muscles of local anaesthetic alone are diagnostic but can be followed by the effective injection of steroid. Skeletal muscle relaxants such as baclofen at a dose of 5 mg three times a day are also used. Local muscle relaxation can be achieved with massage, heat and botulinum toxin. Claims are also made in favour of transcutaneous electrical nerve stimulation (TENS) and acupuncture. Generalized muscle relaxation can be achieved by relaxation therapies and biofeedback techniques. Cognitive strategies that recognize the importance of beliefs that the pain is disabling may be particularly valuable in this population. The effectiveness of antidepressant drugs is demonstrated in controlled trials.

Internal derangement of the temporomandibular joint

This refers to distortion of the anatomy of the joint. Pain is exacerbated by jaw movement. There is swelling and tenderness of the joint and overlying muscles. Joint noises are common.

The cause is usually anterior displacement of the disc as a result of trauma, ligament laxity or changes in the fluid environment of the joint. The condition is not considered further here, since it is predominantly a surgical condition.

Atypical facial pain

In this condition pain tends to be present every day and lasts for most of the day. It can last from hours to months. It is a poorly localized, steady, deep burning or throbbing pain.

It is unrelated to movement. It can migrate and has no anatomically defined distribution. It has no associated physical signs. Provoking or exacerbating factors may be many; little if anything seems to relieve it. Sufferers exhibit depressive features. They are also preoccupied with finding alternative explanations for their conditions. The internet has provided many opportunities for them to enquire and be informed about other diagnoses such as trigeminal neuralgia. It is most common in females over the age of 45 years. Confusingly some authors blur the distinction between it and atypical trigeminal neuralgia.

Treatment

It is most important to identify and treat the large contribution to pain from psychological, social and psychiatric factors. Medical treatment of depression may be necessary, including appropriate doses of antidepressants. Otherwise, the lower doses of antidepressants may be useful. Claims have been made for the combination of tricyclic antidepressant and phenothiazine, also for biofeedback and relaxation techniques and for transcutaneous nerve stimulation.

Facial neuralgias

These refer to trigeminal, glossopharyngeal and nervus intermedius neuralgias. With the exception of trigeminal neuralgia (TGN), they are uncommon. TGN is covered in detail elsewhere in the book.

Glossopharyngeal neuralgia is a milder disease than trigeminal neuralgia, as indicated by the number of episodes, character and treatment of pain. The source of the pain is the anatomical base of the glossopharyngeal nerve (IX cranial nerve). Pain is felt unilaterally in the ear, base of the tongue, tonsils, pharynx or beneath the angle of the jaw. Its pathophysiology and time factors are the same as those for trigeminal neuralgia, but may in addition be associated with syncope. The triggers for glossopharyngeal neuralgia are swallowing, yawning, eating, coughing or talking. Treatment is the same as the conservative treatment of trigeminal neuralgia, although surgical treatments exist (see chapter on trigeminal neuralgia).

(Painful) Trigeminal neuropathy

This describes a peripheral neuropathy involving the named nerve, which may on occasion be painful. There should be a sensory deficit to examination. It can be associated with systemic disease such as diabetes or scleroderma, a structural lesion such as the rare trigeminal schwannoma or medial sphenoid wing meningioma or more usually be idiopathic. Treatment for the pain involves the same medications used for neuropathic pain.

Neuropathic pain following nerve injury

There is no reason why the trigeminal nerve and therefore the face should not suffer the same neuropathic pains that may follow partial injury to the nerve. Typically there will be a dysaesthetic pain sensation, perhaps with allodynia. This can follow facial trauma, which may be surgical – e.g. after base of skull procedures or mastoid operations. Neuromata are common following facial trauma, particularly blow-out orbital fractures and Le Fort III fractures.

Neuropathic pains may complicate base of skull surgery. They are frequently palpated at the site of exit of supraorbital, infraorbital and mental nerves. *Anaesthesia dolorosa* – following neuroablative treatments for trigeminal neuralgia – comes into this category.

Management. Treatment is medical in the first instance – using the usual agents (carbamazepine, gabapentin, antidepressants). Diagnostic local anaesthetic nerve blocks can localize the site of pain, but there are obvious risks (of precipitating further neuropathic pain) if attempts to produce a more permanent nerve block are attempted.

Surgical approaches can be used. High cervical spinal cord stimulation may be successful, and in refractory cases success is claimed in deep brain stimulation and motor cortex stimulation. Trigeminal DREZ (dorsal root entry zone) lesions have been attempted.

Post-herpetic neuralgia

Approximately 4% of patients with herpes zoster will experience pain 1 year after the rash has resolved; this complication is more likely the older the patient, the more severe the rash and acute pain and for females. Treatment is dealt with elsewhere in this book.

Trigeminal autonomic cephalgias

Three conditions are included in this category, but they may not be aetiologically linked. All syndromes involve unilateral autonomic features such as watering of the eye, injection of the cornea, occasionally pupillary changes and ptosis, and hyperaemia of the nasal passages and sinus.

The conditions comprise short-lived unilateral neuralgiform pain with conjunctival tearing (SUNCT), chronic paroxysmal hemicrania (CPH) and cluster headache. For convenience, all are dealt with in the section on headache.

Central post-stroke pain

This syndrome may involve the face, but usually other areas in addition, and there will be an accompaning neurological deficit. It is considered elsewhere in the book.

Differential diagnosis of facial pain

This is a sufficiently important topic to deserve its own section. It is bedevilled by differences in taxonomy – for example between classical trigeminal neuralgia, atypical trigeminal neuralgia and atypical facial pain. The differential diagnosis is dependent almost exclusively on the history, and efforts currently involve trying to determine the key points in the history that will differentiate between syndromes. Then, a hierarchical analysis or diagnostic algorithm can be applied; some workers are attempting to develop a computer-aided diagnostic system based on neural network theory.

The most useful points in the history are the time course of the pain, and its character. Exacerbating and relieving factors are important, as are autonomic features. The presence

Table 1. Differential diagnosis of facial pain

Feature	Classical TGN	Atypical TGN	Atypical facial pain	Trigeminal neuropathy	Cluster headache	CPH	SUNCT	Migraine	PHN	Neuropathic pain; anaesthesia dolorosa
Aetiology	Idiopathic MS Neurovascular compression		Depression	Idiopathic or structural lesion	Trigeminal autonomic cephalgias			Neural dysfunction	Post herpes zoster	Trauma Therapeutic lesion
Time course	Paroxysms Remissions	Paroxysms continuous background Remissions	Continuous	Continuous	15–180 min Relapse and remits	2–45 min	5–240 s	Hours to days Aura Transient neurological deficit	Continuous	Continuous
Alcohol					Triggers	Mild trigger				
Drugs	CBZ	CBZ	Anti-depressants		Triptans	Indometacin	Lamotrigine			
Allodynia									Yes	Yes
Triggering	Yes	Yes								
Autonomic features					Yes	Yes	Yes			

TGN, trigeminal neuralgia; CPH, chronic paroxysmal hemicrania; SUNCT, short-lived unilateral neuralgiform pain; MS, multiple sclerosis; PHN, post-herpetic neuralgia; TMJ, temporomandibular joint; CBZ, carbamazepine.

or absence of allodynia is significant. Again this can confuse – in this account the triggering phenomenon of trigeminal neuralgia is not considered to be a variety of allodynia, though this position is not held universally. Table 1 compares and contrasts the features of the different syndromes in a way that is useful in the differential diagnosis.

Consistency of history is not always present, and it may be necessary to interview the patient on more than one occasion.

Further reading

Classification Committee of the International Headache Society. Classification and diagnostic criteria for head disorders, cranial neuralgias and facial pain. Cephalalgia 2004; 24(Suppl 1): 1–160.

Systematic reviews

Antczak Bouckoms A, Marbach JJ, Glass EG, Glaros AG. Reaction Papers to Chapters 12 and 13. In: Sessle BJ, Bryant PS, Diohne RA, eds. Temporomandibular Disorders and Related Pain Conditions, Vol. 4. Seattle: IASP Press, 1994; 237–45.
Onghena P, Van Houdenhove B. Antidepressant-induced analgesia in chronic non-malignant pain: a meta-analysis of 39 placebo-controlled studies. Pain 1992; 49(2): 205–19.

Related topics of interest

HEADACHE

Headache which is not due to intracranial or systemic pathology is described as primary headache. Primary headaches are appropriately treated in the pain clinic. A working diagnosis of primary headache is made from the history. However, a diagnosis of primary headache can only be entertained after all relevant causes of secondary headache have been excluded. Examination and investigations may be necessary to exclude secondary headache.

Secondary headache: red flags in headache presentation

A comprehensive discussion of secondary headache is impossible as it amounts to an account of intracranial neurosurgery and neurology! Treatment, obviously, is of the cause. However the non-specialist needs to have an idea of which patients need further investigation. A number of features may be regarded as 'red flags', which are symptoms and signs of potentially serious pathology. Imaging or urgent referral to a neurosciences unit is mandatory.

In particular the following should be noted:

- Headache due to tumour or irritation of the dura is suggested by **any** focal neurological deficit either symptomatically or by examination. Typically the headache is novel and progressive in severity over a period of weeks.
  - An organic confusional state should be regarded as a focal sign.
  - Although often cited as a feature of headache of raised intracranial pressure, early morning headache is neither typical nor reliable as a diagnostic feature. Examination must be thorough and include an assessment for papilloedema, and measurement of blood pressure. Included also is an assessment of mental state.
  - Any of these features to which epilepsy – typically focal or 'partial' – may be added should be regarded as an intracranial 'red flag'.
- Chronic headaches which may be present in hydrocephalus or other disturbances of cerebrospinal fluid (CSF) dynamics are extremely complex to manage and can require intracranial pressure monitoring or other studies of CSF dynamics. Obviously management in a neurosciences unit is required.
- Headache of sudden onset requires that vascular causes including subarachnoid haemorrhage be excluded. Although the presentation may be dramatic and obvious, this may not always be the case, and a short-lived transient attack of headache can be a so-called 'warning leak' and is the first presentation in 10–20% of cases of subarachnoid haemorrhage.
- Bitemporal headache, with tenderness and visual failure, especially with tenderness over the artery, requires that the diagnosis of temporal arteritis be excluded. The erythrocyte sedimentation rate (ESR) will be high, and biopsy of the artery may be required. Steroid treatment is needed urgently to preserve vision. Neurological advice should be urgently obtained.

Migraine

Pathophysiology

It is increasingly accepted that migraine is primarily a neural disease and the vascular changes seen are secondary consequences. This hypothesis finds strong support from both positron emission tomography (PET) and functional magnetic resonance imaging (fMRI) studies showing ipsilateral activations in spontaneous and experimentally triggered migraine (by sublingual glycerol trinitrate) in the dorsolateral pons. These changes are not seen in other primary headaches such as cluster headache or chronic paroxysmal hemicrania. In addition there is a genetic predisposition with specific gene loci identified in specific situations, e.g. familial hemiplegic migraine. It is a common condition, and as many as 15% of the population may experience attacks at one time or another.

Separate theories of vascular and neural mechanisms of physiology have been proposed to explain the mechanism of headache. The two mechanisms may act together, with calcitonin gene-related peptide (CGRP) playing a central role as a neurotransmitter with vasodilating activity.

Experimental work has been limited because of the absence of an animal model on which hypotheses and drugs can be tested. Agonists for a subtype of 5-hydroxytryptamine receptor known as 5HT1 agonists have been useful. The 5HT1 receptor has its own subpopulation of receptors, one of which, known as 5HT1δ, is involved in the mechanism of CGRP action.

Diagnosis

Diagnostic criteria have been described by the Headache Classification Committee of the International Headache Society. Migraine is classified as migraine without aura and migraine with aura (classical migraine). The former is more common.

Diagnostic criteria for migraine without aura

1. At least five attacks fulfilling criteria 2–4.
2. Headache lasts 4–72 hours, untreated or unsuccessfully treated.
3. Headache has at least two of the following characteristics:
   - Unilateral location.
   - Pulsating quality.
   - Moderate or severe intensity (inhibits or prohibits daily activities).
   - Aggravation by routine physical activity.
4. During headache at least one of the following:
   - Nausea and/or vomiting.
   - Photophobia and phonophobia.

History, examination and/or investigation must exclude another disorder which could account for the headache. If such a disorder is present, diagnosis of migraine requires that attacks do not occur for the first time in close temporal relation to that disorder.

Premonitory symptoms can occur before an attack of migraine without aura. They usually consist of hyper- or hypoactivity, depression, craving for particular foods or repetitive yawning.

Aura is a complex of neurological symptoms which can initiate or accompany an attack. Symptoms may be localized to the cerebral cortex or brain stem. Typical aura are visual disturbances, sensory symptoms, weakness or dysphasia. Migraine aura can be unaccompanied by headache.

Migraine can be triggered by factors such as stress, withdrawal from caffeine, dietary factors such as the ingestion of chocolate, cheese, wines and seafood, and hormonal changes due to the menstrual cycle or hormonal medication. Stress and hormonal factors are each identified triggers in 60% of migraine sufferers. Dietary factors have been implicated in approximately 20%. Frequently there is a family history of migraine.

Management

Management is by prevention of attacks and intermittent treatment of attacks. The choice between prophylactic therapy and the sole use of abortive treatments depends on the frequency, severity and impact of acute attacks.

Prophylaxis

Drug therapy used for prevention aims to reduce the frequency of attacks by 50% and to reduce the severity of attacks when they do occur. The effect of the drug on the headache and its associated symptoms should be closely monitored. All drugs have side effects and their benefits need to be accurately compared to their disadvantages. Explanation and reassurance reduce the incidence and severity of attacks. Patients should be educated to avoid triggers where possible.

- *β-Blockers* (for example, propranolol 80–240 mg daily in divided doses). Propranolol has been shown to induce a 43% reduction in migraine headache activity. When improvements were assessed using further outcomes, they were found to be 20% greater. Propranolol 160 mg daily yielded a 44% reduction in migraine activity when daily headache recordings were used to assess outcome. With less-conservative outcome measures there was a 65% reduction in migraine activity. β-Blockers are thought to have some activity at 5HT subreceptors.
- *Sodium valproate* has been shown to be effective in reducing frequency of migraine by 50% over a 12-week period. The combined number needed to treat (NNT) for 3 trials was 3.5.
- *Pizotifen* is a 5HT antagonist that has been shown to confer a prophylactic benefit in patients who take sumatriptan for acute treatment of symptoms. Pizotifen does not alter the severity of migraine. Its proven effect therefore is one of reducing the use of sumatriptan. Its principal side effect is weight gain.
- *Miscellaneous drugs* Nimodipine, clonidine and fluoxitene are not effective in the prophylaxis of migraine.

The difficulty with drug prophylaxis, the potential side effects and a require-ment to take the drugs constantly has generated much interest in non-pharma-cological methods, of which the following are notable:

- **Relaxation** and **biofeedback training** have been shown to be of benefit.
- **Occlusal splinting devices** have been shown to reduce the frequency and duration of migraine. A trial design used a 'placebo' intraoral device that covered the palatal mucosa but did not alter the mechanics of occlusion.
- **Occipital nerve stimulation** is currently under investigation – there is positive evidence from controlled observations.

Treatment of attacks

Evidence from randomized controlled trials supports:

- **Triptans** Sumatriptan is a 5HT1δ agonist. Its major advantages are rapid onset and high efficacy. Given orally at a dose of 50 or 100 mg the attack is relieved in half to two-thirds of patients. If the symptoms are not relieved a subsequent dose should not be taken. If symptoms are relieved but later recur a further dose can be taken, up to a maximum of 300 mg in 24 hours. The subcutaneous injection of 6 mg relieves 88% of attacks and may be useful if attacks are of rapid onset. Headache settles in approximately 30 minutes. Sumatriptan should be used with caution in patients with a history of cardiovascular disease. Alternative triptans include rizatriptan 10 mg, almotriptan 12.5 mg, eletriptan 40 mg or zolmitriptan 2.5 mg

In addition reports of success with the following have been made:

- **Paracetamol with metoclopramide.**
- **Nonsteroidal anti-inflammatory drugs (NSAIDs)** can be effective. They are given with antiemetics to treat a relatively mild attack. They have the advan-tage of being available in parenteral and suppository forms should nausea occur and preclude the oral route.
- **Biofeedback techniques, hypnosis and acupuncture** have also been used for the treatment of acute attacks. They are best used early.
- **Ergotamine** is given as a dose of 2 mg initially, repeated with 1 mg to a maximum of 5 mg. It is a powerful vasoconstrictor and should not be given to those with peripheral, cerebral or coronary vascular disease, nor to the pregnant patient or the known drug abuser.

Trigeminal autonomic cephalgias

A variety of conditions are placed in this category which comprises cluster headache; chronic paroxysmal headache and short-lived unilateral neuralgiform pain with conjuncti-val tearing. Although an aetiology is implied by this categorization, it remains unproven. Migraine is sometimes, though innappropriately, included in this category.

Cluster headache

This condition is otherwise known as migrainous neuralgia or Horton's syndrome, although its aetiology is not now considered as equivalent to migraine. The posterior hypothalamus has been implicated in structural MRI studies using voxel-based morphometry, and activations in PET studies. This contrasts with areas of activation found in migraine (see above). The term derives from the fact that the attacks are clustered in time and space.

Diagnostic criteria

1. At least five attacks fulfilling criteria 2–4.
2. Severe unilateral orbital, supraorbital and/or temporal pain lasting 15–180 minutes untreated.
3. Headache is associated with at least one of the following signs, which have to be present on the same side as the pain:
   - Conjunctival injection.
   - Lacrimation.
   - Nasal congestion.
   - Rhinorrhoea.
   - Forehead and facial sweating.
   - Miosis.
   - Ptosis.
   - Eyelid oedema.
4. Frequency of attacks: from one every other day to eight per day.

History, examination and investigation must exclude another disorder which might account for the pain, or if such a disorder is present cluster headache should not occur for the first time in close temporal relation to the disorder.

Cluster headache occurs predominantly in men, in the fourth decade of life. Attacks occur in 'clusters' lasting 4–10 weeks. Most commonly they happen two to three times a day. Bouts of headaches often occur in early spring or early autumn. Clusters are interspersed by pain-free periods of months to years, but rarely more than 2 years. Headaches usually last about 45 minutes. They can occur at any time of day but typically start soon after the onset of sleep. The pain is burning in character. Classically sufferers have deep nasolabial folds and *peau d'orange* skin changes. Precipitating factors include alcohol and altitude. Typically attacks may be triggered by alcohol, and during an attack the victim finds it impossible to keep still.

Management

Management may be directed either against an acute attack or be prophylactic.

Acute attacks

- Triptans: may need intranasal or intramuscular administration.
- 100% oxygen by inhalation.
- A short course of prednisolone.

Prophylactic treatments

- Abstinence from alcohol.
- Verapamil 40–80 mg three times a day
- Prednisolone.
- Ergotamine 1–2 mg rectally before the attack.
- Methysergide 2 mg three times a day
- Lithium.
- Sphenopalatine local anaesthetic block.
- Sphenopalatine ganglion radiofrequency lesions.
- Partial trigeminal nerve ablation.
- Deep brain stimulation.
- Occipital nerve stimulation

In severe cases surgical treatments have been attempted, including foramen ovale lesioning of the trigeminal nerve as might be done in trigeminal neuralgia. Recently, after abnormalities were identified in the ipsilateral posterior hypothalamus by voxel-based MRI morphometry, this has been used as a target for deep brain stimulation. Less invasively, stimulation of the occipital nerve is also under trial for this condition.

Short-lived unilateral neuralgiform pain with conjunctival tearing

Short-lived unilateral neuralgiform pain with conjunctival tearing (SUNCT) is extremely rare. It occurs typically in elderly men. Treatment can be extremely difficult, but some success has been obtained with lamotrigine.

Chronic paroxysmal hemicrania

Chronic paroxysmal hemicrania (CPH) has the same features as cluster headache but attacks occur 15–20 times a day and last 3–15 minutes. It is more common in women and does not follow the onset of sleep. The aetiology is unknown. Treatment is indometacin 75–150 mg orally and the response is diagnostic. Verapamil has been used as a prophylactic agent.

Tension headache

Diagnostic critera

1. At least 10 previous headache episodes, with frequency less than 180 headaches per year or less than 15 per month.
2. Headaches lasting 30 minutes to 7 days.
3. At least two of the following:
   - Pressing, tightening, non-pulsating.
   - Mild or moderate.
   - Bilateral.
   - No aggravation by routine physical activity.

4. Both of the following:
   - No nausea or vomiting; anorexia may occur.
   - Never both photophobia and phonophobia.

History, examination and investigation must exclude another disorder which might account for pain, or if such a disorder is present tension headache must not occur for the first time in close temporal relation to the disorder.

Headaches usually occur daily. There is a history of stress, and depression may coexist. It is more common in women. Overuse of analgesics aggravates the situation. Examination may reveal tender points.

Management

Depression should be treated if necessary. Small doses of tricyclic antidepressants are also effective in patients without clear signs of depression. Otherwise, benefit has been claimed with relaxation and cognitive strategies and NSAIDs.

Cervicogenic headache

This is headache which originates in the structures in the neck. Pain from one or both sides of the neck radiates to the occiput, temples or frontal area. It is a dull pain, worse in the morning and exacerbated by movement or tension. Lateral flexion and rotational movements are restricted. Headache is often due to irritation of the C2 and C3 nerve roots and the greater occipital nerve.

Management

Steroid injections to cervical facet joints gives temporary relief in 60–70% of patients. Benefit has also been claimed for greater occipital nerve blocks, transcutaneous electrical nerve stimulation (TENS), acupuncture and physiotherapy. There is now evidence that occipital nerve stimulation may be effective in this condition.

Occipital neuralgia

This is a paroxysmal jabbing pain in the distribution of the greater or lesser occipital nerves. Aching can persist between paroxysms and there may be altered sensation. The affected nerve is tender to palpation.

The pain is eased temporarily by local anaesthetic block of the appropriate nerve. Subsequent injections of steroid are claimed to be of benefit. The use of occipital nerve stimulation has also been tried with success.

Analgesic headache

Large daily doses of aspirin, paracetamol or weak opioids taken for the treatment of headache can aggravate headache. The daily use of ergotamine for headache or sudden withdrawal from ergotamine induces headache. The withdrawal headache is thought to be due to vasodilatory counteracting mechanisms which have developed during the use of the drug but are left unopposed when the drug is withdrawn. Sumatriptan, used for the treatment of migraine, causes the same problems. Admission for 'detoxification' – withdrawal of analgesics – may be needed in extreme cases.

Management

Recommendations for prevention are:

- Analgesics should not be taken every day for the treatment of headaches.
- Ergotamine should not be taken more than 10 times a month.
- There should be restrictions on the use of sumatriptan, to approximately 10 times a month.
- Opioid drugs should not be used for the treatment of headache.

Miscellaneous headaches

A number of primary headaches do not fit into these specific categories, such as those provoked by physical exertion, sexual activity, certain foods, very cold foods, coughing or restricting devices worn on the head. Avoidance of provoking factors should be advised where possible. NSAIDs are reported to be of value.

Further reading

Classification Committee of the International Headache Society. Classification and diagnostic criteria for head disorders, cranial neuralgia and facial pain. Cephalalgia 2004; 24(Suppl 1): 1–160.

Connor HE. The aetiology of headache. Pain Reviews 1994; 1(2):77–88.

Goadsby PJ. Recent advances in the diagnosis and management of migraine. British Medical Journal 2006; 332: 25–9.

Olesen J. Analgesic headache. British Medical Journal 1997; 310: 479–80.

Systematic review

Onghena P, Van Houdenhove B. Antidepressant-induced analgesia in chronic non-malignant pain: a meta-analysis of 39 placebo-controlled studies. Pain 1992; 49(2): 205–19.

Related topics of interest

Depression and pain (p. 69); Facial pain (p. 73).

IMMUNODEFICIENCY DISEASE AND PAIN

Acquired immune deficiency syndrome (AIDS)

The acquired immune deficiency syndrome is a painful disease. Not only is there a high incidence of patients reporting pain but also some two-thirds of all patients describe constant pain interfering with their lives to a significant or severe degree. Many different pain syndromes are described, and patients present with more than one, said to be an average of three different pains. Not only is pain in AIDS inadequately treated but it also threatens to pose a greater problem as survival rates improve.

Pain is due to disease or treatment. The pain profile is unique to the disease. There are significant psychological and social consequences of disease which have a bearing on the pain syndrome, complex medication of antiretroviral therapy and treatment and prophylaxis for opportunistic infections and cancers. Sufferers may be substance abusers, which adds further complexity to the management of the condition. Patients are at increased risk of infection and neoplastic disorders and this should be borne in mind when providing symptomatic treatment.

Pain due to disease can be:

1. Gastrointestinal
- Oral and oesophageal candidiasis.
- Dental abscess.
- Aphthous ulceration.
- Mouth ulceration due to cytomegalovirus and herpes virus infection.
- Necrotizing gingivitis.
- Oesophageal ulceration.
- Gastrointestinal cramps associated with *Shigella*, *Salmonella* and *Campylobacter* infection.
- Small bowel obstruction and perforation, small bowel lymphoma.
- Cytomegalovirus colitis.
- Spontaneous peritonitis.
- Cholecystitis or cholangitis due to *Cryptosporidium* or cytomegalovirus infection.
- Proctitis and perianal abscess.

2. Neurological
- Brain tumour.
- Encephalitis.
- Aseptic meningitis.
- Cerebral toxoplasmosis.
- Cryptococcal meningitis.
- Painful symmetrical neuropathy due to direct action of HIV virus on peripheral nerves (affect approximately a quarter of patients).

- Cytomegalovirus infection of dorsal root ganglion.
- Demyelinating polyneuropathy.

3. Rheumatological
- Reiter's syndrome.
- Sacroiliitis
- Polyarthralgia associated with mononucleosis.
- Psoriasis and psoriatic arthropathy.
- Reactive arthritis.
- Polymyositis.

4. Tumour
- Kaposi's sarcoma.

5. Pain due to treatment
- Pancreatitis is a consequence of retroviral therapy.
- Indinavir urolithiasis causing renal colic – requires hydration, narcotics and temporary cessation. If intervention is necessary, endoscopic stent placement may be needed.
- Antivirals, antimicrobials and *Pneumocystis carinii* prophylaxis.
- Chemotherapy reaction, surgery procedures, bronchoscopies, biopsies.

The principles of pain assessment and management are not fundamentally different from those with cancer and justify the input of many professionals. Treatment may be pharmacological, anaesthetic, psychotherapeutic, and spiritual issues may have to be addressed also.

As far as analgesic management is concerned, the analgesic ladder is an accepted method of titrating drug potency to symptoms but due consideration must be given to the requirement for treatments for neuropathic pain and the use of psychotropic agents. Of interest is the requirement for opioids in patients with a prior history of opioid abuse. Patients may be tolerant of opioids, or anxious about using them. The principles of pain management in such patients include an acceptance that opioids may be appropriate, that there may be a potential for abuse, but more importantly that adequate pain relief cannot be withheld because of fears of potential abuse.

Further reading

Larue F, Fontaine A, Colleau SM. Underestimation and undertreatment of pain in HIV disease: multi-centre study. British Medical Journal 1997; 314: 23–9.
O'Neil W, Sherrard JS. Pain in human immunodeficiency disease: a review. Pain 1993; 54: 3–14.

Related topics of interest

Cancer pain – drugs (p. 50); Therapy – opioids in chronic pain (p. 224).

IRRITABLE BOWEL AND OESOPHAGEAL PAIN

This chapter considers painful disorders of the digestive tract including irritable bowel syndrome and non-ulcer dyspepsia. Differential diagnosis between the latter and non-cardiac chest pain (dealt with in a separate chapter) may be very difficult; both are usefully considered as visceral pain syndromes with common features.

Anatomy/physiology of visceral pain

Primary afferent nociceptive fibres enter the spinal cord via fibres which pass with efferent nerves of both the sympathetic (thoracic and lumbar spinal nerve roots) and parasympathetic (sacral nerve roots) divisions of the autonomic nervous system.

The viscera are innervated by a population of C fibres which are refractory to stimulation unless sensitized by pathological processes (silent nociceptors).

There is poor localization of visceral pain due to the wide receptive fields for dorsal horn cells receiving input from visceral afferents. Localization of pain requires stimulation of the parietal peritoneum.

Irritable bowel syndrome

Irritable bowel syndrome (IBS) presents as crampy lower abdominal pain associated with either frequent loose stools or infrequent hard stools. Associated, distressing symptoms include bloating and a sensation of incomplete rectal emptying. Patients may complain of either diarrhoea or constipation.

The prolonged contractions of the colon which are suspected as being the major physiological alteration of IBS can be provoked by emotional factors. Stressful life events and a history of sexual abuse are worth noting as predisposing factors. IBS also occurs as a complication of infection of the gastrointestinal tract. The abnormal mechanoreceptor activation associated with a prolonged contraction may result in sensitization of primary afferents, and an exaggerated response to normally innocuous stimulation. This theory explains tenderness of the colon during palpation, and pain and spasm of bowel distension during sigmoidoscopy. The pain is therefore one of mechanical allodynia and hyperalgesia of viscera to non-painful and painful stimuli, respectively. The mechanism may be either one of primary afferent and dorsal horn sensitization or reduction of tonic supraspinal inhibition of autonomic afferent activity. It is possible that both mechanisms are acting, leading to a 'positive feedback' loop in which peripheral afferents become increasingly sensitized by removal of supraspinal inhibition. More severe cases of IBS complain of constant symptoms that are not relieved by the passage of stool.

Non-cardiac chest pain and non-ulcer dyspepsia

Non-cardiac chest pain may account for up to 30% of admissions to coronary care units, and in view of the seriousness of the differential diagnosis of cardiac chest pain, may commit the physician to expensive, and risky, investigation (for example, coronary angiography). Abnormalities of oesophageal peristalsis and acid reflux may be responsible for pain in some cases, but there remains a group where neither of these account for the pain. This group of patients may have abnormalities of muscle regulation of oesophageal diameter associated with visceral hyperalgesia. Non-ulcer dyspepsia is therefore an analogous visceral pain syndrome to irritable bowel syndrome in the upper gastrointestinal tract.

Management

Psychological approaches, particularly methods involving relaxation, have a role in the management of all these conditions. Explanation of the cause of the condition may reassure the patient who is convinced of the serious nature of the condition, and seeks reassurance from repeated examination or endoscopy. The following account of therapies of the various syndromes is not exhaustive:

- *Hypnotherapy* has been shown to work in IBS.
- *Ispaghula husk and propantheline* has been shown to relieve symptoms of IBS and maintain remission.
- *Cognitive therapy* has been shown to reduce gastrointestinal symptoms in IBS.
- *Loperamide* has been shown to reduce overall pain intensity, but at the expense of increased night pain.
- *Cromoglycate and antihistamines (ketanserin and H$_2$ blockers)* have been claimed as effective drugs in the treatment of post-infectious IBS.
- *Antidepressants* have been claimed to be effective in IBS.
- *Smooth muscle relaxants* such as *glyceryl trinitrate, hydralazine, nifedipine* and *diltiazem* have been described for treatment of non-cardiac chest pain. The mode of action is believed to be on the muscle of the oesophagus. That these drugs act also on the heart may lead to difficulties in diagnosis.

Further reading

Mayer EA, Munakata J, Mertz H, Lembo T, Bernstein CN. Visceral hyperalgesia and irritable bowel syndrome. In: Gebhardt GF, ed. Visceral Pain, Progress in Pain Research and Management, Vol. 5. Seattle: IASP Press, 1995; 429–68.

Related topic of interest

Chest pain (p. 56).

MULTIPLE SCLEROSIS

Multiple sclerosis (MS) is a progressive disease. It is characterized by initial destruction of myelin and eventually axons and cell bodies. It can affect any part of the central nervous system (CNS). It is well established that MS is a painful condition. There are varying reports of the incidence of pain such as:

- 40% of MS patients are never pain-free.
- 64% report pain at some time of their disease.
- 48% have more than one pain.
- 32% of pain sufferers with MS rate pain amongst the most severe symptoms of their disease.
- Prevalence of pain for the preceding month has been quoted at 53%.

Pain can be:

- Disease related.
- Disability related.

There should be routine assessment for pain in MS patients, with attention given to each pain.

Disease-related pain

Pain related to the disease tends to occur when the disease is well established, although 23% have pain at the time of onset of the disease. The proportion of time in pain increases with disease severity, but pain intensity does not increase with disease severity. The number of people in pain increases with disease duration. Of those in pain, 44% have difficulty sleeping and 34% have difficulty with personal relationships. Pain results in poorer mental health and increased social handicap. Pain from MS is predominant in females at a ratio higher than the female predominance of MS itself. The incidence of pain due to MS increases with age.

Pain peculiar to MS sufferers is of two types.

Persistent neuropathic pain

Persistent pain occurs in an estimated 17–66% of MS patients. Lesions anywhere in the CNS may be the cause of pain but lesions of the spinal cord, lower brain stem and periventricular areas of the forebrain are more likely to be the cause. Although the demyelinating process of MS causes conduction block, secondary reorganization of membrane electrical properties occurs, causing hyperexcitability and pain.

Pain tends to be extensive. It frequently affects the legs but can occur in more than one area. It is often described as burning and demonstrates allodynia and hyperalgesia. Visceral afferents can affect pain.

Intermittent pain

Intermittent pain is experienced as:

- Spasms and tonic seizures – more likely to occur if spasticity is uncontrolled.
- Tightening painful sensations of the extremities.
- Trigeminal and glossopharyngeal neuralgias – these may be caused by demyelination of the brain stem. Trigeminal neuralgia occurs in up to 5% of MS sufferers. It differs from primary trigeminal neuralgia in that there is a constant background of pain with superimposed spasms of pain, typical of classical trigeminal neuralgia, it occurs in a younger population, and is more likely to be bilateral. Of those with bilateral trigeminal neuralgia, 18% have MS. In addition there are paroxysms of pain similar to those of classical trigeminal neuralgia.
- L'Hermitte's sign. This sign refers to the occurrence of an electrical sensation passing down the back to the legs on flexion of the neck. It is reported at some time in up to 25% of MS patients. It is related to disease involving the dorsal columns and cervical nerve roots. It is not always painful.
- Abdominal pain. This is thought to be neuropathic and occurs in 2% of sufferers.
- A girdle or radicular distribution occurring acutely in the absence of obvious nerve compression. This may be due to demyelination of root entry zones and is perceived as burning pain.

Disability-related pain

Musculoskeletal pains

These are caused by postural and musculoskeletal abnormalities arising from paresis, spasms, discoordination and immobility.

Low back pain increases with disease duration. Approximately 39% have low back pain.

Peripheral neuropathic pains

Nerve compression secondary to musculoskeletal deformities can cause neuropathic pain.

Although depressive symptoms and cognitive disturbances are recognized in MS sufferers, the incidence of such symptoms does not differ between MS sufferers with pain and MS sufferers without pain.

Management

Each pain must be dealt with separately, albeit that treatment of more than one pain may be achieved by a single pharmacological tool. Attention must be given to associated symptoms of psychological distress.

The general principles of treatment of neuropathic pain are applied to the persistent pain, the neuralgias, optic neuritis, sometimes to the abdominal pain and to neuropathic pain arising from disability.

Treatment should start with the tricyclic antidepressants with anticonvulsants as second line of treatment. Gabapentin and lamotrigine have been reported to be of use.

Treatment of pain due to spasm, tonic seizures and spasticity has been the subject of many controlled trials. Unfortunately, few trials used a reliable and validated measurement of spasticity such as the Ashworth Scoring System.

Gabapentin proved effective over a 48-hour period and was then chosen and used for long-term therapy in one trial. Other drugs used in trials, but described in a systematic review as lacking in adequate methods for measuring spasticity, include baclofen, dantrolene, tizanidine, botulinum toxin, vigabatrin, prazepam and threonine. Reports claim the benefit of carbamazepine. There are reports as to the effectiveness of cannabis lasting several hours after administration. Reports of mexiletine effectiveness are tempered by suspicion that paralysis may appear to worsen. There is excellent evidence for the efficacy of intrathecal baclofen in the management of spasticity and the pain resulting from spasticity.

Trigeminal neuralgia

Although surgical treatment for primary trigeminal neuralgia in the operation of microvascular decompression is effective, this is not so for trigeminal neuralgia due to MS, where the characteristic pathology of primary trigeminal neuralgia is absent. Trigeminal neuralgia secondary to MS is shown to be best treated with anticonvulsant drugs, the most popular choice being carbamazepine. Five out of six patients treated with topiramate 25 mg twice daily increasing by 50 mg per week up to a maximum of 200 mg twice daily had complete relief. There are also reports of the success of percutaneous retrogasserian glycerol rhizotomy (reports of 38–88% complete relief) and radiofrequency lesioning of the ganglion. Glossopharyngeal neuralgia associated with MS responds to carbamezepine.

L'Hermitte's sign

L'Hermitte's sign pain is said to respond to weak electromagnetic fields but this is not a widely available treatment.

Abdominal pain

Abdominal pain may be treated by sympathetic blockade using local anaesthetic alone. This technique may provide pain relief beyond the pharmacological duration of the local anaesthetic.

Musculoskeletal pain

Physiotherapy assessment is valuable for determining the relative contribution of the musculoskeletal system to the presentation of pain, and for the supply of appropriate appliances and local treatments. Standard analgesics, including anti-inflammatory drugs where appropriate, may also be of value. Transcutaneous electrical nerve stimulation (TENS) and acupuncture may be of value if the cutaneous sensation is preserved, but may be ineffective, even poorly tolerated, if the nerve pathways from primary afferent large-diameter fibres are affected by the disease process. As in any case presenting with low back pain, sinister pathology and surgically operable lesions must be excluded.

Treatment may be difficult, as provoking factors are likely to persist. Radicular pain can be treated by drugs effective for neuropathic pain. Epidural steroids may be considered, but there is a potential medicolegal hazard in using a drug without a product licence on a central nervous system suffering from an unpredictable and progressive disease.

Further reading

Clifford DB, Trotter JL. Pain in multiple sclerosis. Archives of Neurology 1984; 41: 1270–2.
Kassirer MR, Osterberg DH. Pain in chronic multiple sclerosis. Journal of Pain and Symptom Management 1987; 2(2): 95–7.
Stenager E, Knudsen L, Jensen K. Acute and chronic pain syndromes in multiple sclerosis. Acta Neurologica Scandinavica 1991; 84: 197–200.

Systematic review

McQuay H, Carroll D, Jadad AR, Wiffen P, Moore A. Anticonvulsant drugs for the management of pain: a systematic review. British Medical Journal 1995; 311: 1047–52.
Shakespeare DT, Young CA, Boggild M. Antispasticity treatments for multiple sclerosis. The Cochrane Library, Issue 4, 2000. Oxford: Update software.

Related topics of interest

Back pain – injections (p. 28); Facial pain (p. 73); Therapy – anticonvulsants (p. 207); Therapy – antidepressants (p. 209); Therapy – cannabinoids (p. 217).

MUSCULOSKELETAL PAIN SYNDROMES

Joint pain is a presenting feature of many conditions outside the scope of this textbook. Where pain is associated with synovitis and progressive articular cartilage destruction, there is a clear requirement that treatment of the disease process is a key part of the management of pain and the reduction of disability. Pain is to a large extent nociceptive, with the additional factor that chronic nociceptive states induce a permanent state of hyperexcitability of the central nervous system, and chronically painful conditions cause secondary changes in mental well-being and function. The specific management of conditions in which inflammation is part of the disease process will not be discussed here. The reader is referred to rheumatology textbooks for details of the management of rheumatoid arthritis, ankylosing spondylitis, polymyalgia rheumatica and gout. It is worth noting, however, that the disease process of rheumatoid arthritis can be affected by the central nervous system. Thus, rheumatoid arthritis is not observed in joints of a limb affected by a stroke. Palindromic arthritis, a type of rheumatoid arthritis with flitting joint pains and inflammation, has been claimed to respond to block of the sympathetic system.

The musculoskeletal pain syndromes to be discussed here include the syndromes termed fibromyalgia and myofascial pain syndrome, together with conditions associated with a painful shoulder. In these conditions the pain and disability may be considered part of a pain syndrome rather than the result of a progressive nociceptive process. Non-specific low back pain has many features in common with these syndromes.

Fibromyalgia and myofascial pain

The syndromes have as common features symptoms of regional or widespread tenderness. The validity of using separate diagnostic criteria, implying distinct pathology, is questionable. There is a risk that, in focusing on specific pain complaints in the search for symptom relief, the strategy of reducing disability will be ignored. Some authorities have considered the concept of a condition such as fibromyalgia so unhelpful that they have suggested an alternative name, the 'irritable everything syndrome'. One interpretation is that musculoskeletal pain syndromes are overlapping syndromes, variants of muscle pains that otherwise healthy individuals suffer.

Definitions

Given the limitations above, attempts to define individual syndromes are as follows:

Fibromyalgia. Widespread pain: this means bilateral pain, and pain below and above the waist, in addition to neck or back pain.

Pain on digital palpation, using a standard force (4 kg) in 11 of 18 possible sites. The sites are described bilaterally in the following positions and are by convention referred to as 'tender points':

- Suboccipital muscle insertions.
- Anterior aspect of transverse process C5–C7.
- Midpoint of upper border of trapezius.
- On the medial border of the spine of the scapula.
- Costochondral junction of second rib.
- Distal to the lateral epicondyle.
- The upper outer quadrant of the buttock.
- Posterior to the greater trochanter of femur.
- Medial aspect of lower end of femur.

Three-quarters of patients with tenderness in 11 or more of these sites complain of fatigue, sleep disturbance or morning stiffness, and over half complain of headache or pain 'all over'. Sleep disturbance, as described in association with tender points and widespread pain, has particular electrophysiological features.

Myofascial pain syndrome. There is no requirement for the pain to be widespread. Areas where pain is experienced on palpation are, by convention, called trigger points. Trigger points are specific for particular muscles. Pain is experienced in a characteristic regional distribution when trigger points are stimulated. Trigger points are described as occurring within one area of a taut band of muscle fibres, which if snapped in a transverse direction is associated with a local twitch response.

Pathophysiology

It has not proved possible to identify a peripheral source of abnormal noci-ceptor activity in these conditions, although attractive theories concerning metabolic origins for areas of taut muscle fibres abound. Histological and biochemical studies have so far failed to prove these theories. Lowering of threshold to electrical stimulation is not restricted to tender or trigger points identified clinically, but is part of a widespread disorder, and therefore one of central processing.

Management

The following symptoms should alert to the possibility of serious or systemic disease, for example inflammatory arthritis and temporal arteritis:

- Morning stiffness.
- Tenderness over the superficial temporal artery.
- Joint tenderness or swelling.

Regional pain may be perceived in the referred dermatomal distribution of visceral pathology, persisting after the visceral problem has ceased to be a medical problem. Where there is history of trauma, consideration should be given to the spectrum of disorders known as 'complex regional pain syndrome'. Trigger points can be treated with precise needling of the point. The nature of any substance injected is less important than the mechanical disruption of the taut band that is achieved by needling. Local anaesthetic, steroids and neurolytic substances have their advocates. Longitudinal stretching of taut bands can be performed by the therapist or the patient. However, symptom control is no more important than advice about exercise and posture to prevent recurrence.

The evidence for any particular treatment of fibromyalgia syndrome is difficult to assess. The diversity of symptoms and the number of potential outcome measurements that could be made mean that it is difficult to interpret the data from randomized controlled trials. There is no consensus for the use of particular outcome measures: one of the more popular measures, a simple physician-rated scale of global improvement, demonstrates improvement in several drug trials. A systematic review commented that the use of amitriptyline is supported by two out of four randomized controlled trials, using measures of patient-reported pain, physician-reported pain and patient overall (global) assessment, and two out of three trials assessing patients' sleep.

Formal psychosocial and functional assessment with appropriate cognitive/behavioural approaches may be required for patients who do not respond to the measures outlined above.

Frozen shoulder

There is no accepted definition of frozen shoulder and there is no well-defined pathophysiological process. It may be due to scarring in the capsule surrounding the joint. Symptoms are pain and severe restriction of active and passive movement, particularly external rotation. Frozen shoulder affects 2% of adults, usually in the 40–60 years age group. In 20% it subsequently develops in the other shoulder. It is described as having three phases:

- Initial phase is the development of pain over 2–9 months. Pain is worse at night.
- Pain subsides over the subsequent 4–12 months but stiffness and restriction of movement persist.
- The third phase lasts 5–24 months and during this time pain and stiffness resolve.

The course can, however, take much longer and even when symptoms have resolved there can be some limitation in movement. Important conditions such as tendonitis, tears of rotator cuff, arthritis, joint infection, locked posterior dislocation of the glenohumeral joint and systemic disorders must be excluded. Tears of the cuff and tendonitis cause pain and restriction of active movement but not of passive movement as does frozen shoulder. Investigation of these disease entities includes full blood count, erythrocyte sedimentation rate, rheumatoid factor and shoulder X-ray.

Treatments

The authors of a systematic review concluded that the effects of treatment were few.

- **Nonsteroidal anti-inflammatory drugs (NSAIDs).** A systematic review showed these drugs were better than placebo in relieving pain and improving function when used for a few weeks.
- **Corticosteroid injections.** Steroids are injected into the subacromial bursa and into the joint itself. The injection of 20 mg of methylprednisolone in

0.5 ml of 1% lidocaine three times weekly has been shown to improve mobility over the first 4 weeks but not in 2 weeks beyond that. A comparison between 40 mg of methylprednisolone with lidocaine or lidocaine alone has failed to show a difference. Three injections of triamcinolone 40 mg over 6 weeks has been shown to be superior to physiotherapy in improving pain and disability.

- *Oral steroids.* Ten mg prednisolone daily for 4 weeks followed by 5 mg daily for 2 weeks with movement exercises has been shown to be superior to exercise alone for the first few weeks but there is no difference at 5 months.
- *Physiotherapy* includes mobilization, ultrasound, laser, transcutaneous electrical nerve stimulation (TENS), magnet treatment, cold therapy and exercises. It has been shown that exercise is superior to analgesia alone in improving movement and superior to intra-articular triamcinolone alone in improving pain and mobility.
- *Suprascapular nerve block* of 10 ml of 0.5% bupivacaine three times at 7-day intervals alone has been shown to produce reduction in pain 2 weeks after the injection.
- *Manipulation under anaesthesia* has been reported to bring about good improvement but there was no statistical analysis of the data in the trial.

Systematic review

Green S, Buchbinder R, Glazier R, Forbes A. Interventions for shoulder pain (Cochrane review). The Cochrane Library, Issue 4, 2000. Oxford: Update software.

Van der Windt DAWM, van der Heidjen GJMG, Scholten RJPM, Koes BW, Bouter LM. The efficacy of NSAIDs for shoulder complaints. A systematic review. Journal of Clinical Epidemiology 1995; 48: 691–704.

White KP, Harth M. An analytical review of 24 controlled trials for fibromyalgia syndrome. Pain 1996; 64: 211–17.

Related topics of interest

Anatomy and physiology (p. 5); Back pain – medical management (p. 34); Osteoarthritis (p. 166); Therapy – anti-inflammatory drugs (p. 211).

NECK PAIN

Painful neck syndromes are a heterogeneous group of conditions in which many mechanisms may be acting, but in which attention has in particular been directed to two sites of possible pathology: these are the cervical discs and the facet joints. The use of diagnostic nerve blocks has allowed the relative contribution of each site to persistent pain to be determined. In addition to pain arising from joints or discs, there may be muscular pain and pain due to irritation or compression of the cervical or brachial plexus. Secondary hyperalgesia may complicate the clinical presentation and make the precise diagnosis of origin of pain very difficult. Other conditions such as the musculoskeletal pain syndromes and headache syndromes include neck pain amongst the symptoms.

Cervical spine trauma and pain

Pain after cervical spine trauma is typically seen as a consequence of a rear-end impact in a road traffic impact, where it is colloquially termed a 'whiplash' injury. It is estimated that some 20% of victims subjected to this mechanism of injury will develop symptoms. The principal symptom is of pain in the back of the neck that is worsened by movement and may radiate to the head, shoulder, arm or interscapular region. The headache is suboccipital and radiates anteriorly. There may be other symptoms suggestive but not necessarily diagnostic of a somatoform pain disorder. Psychological symptoms amounting to post-traumatic stress disorder may reflect the severe psychological trauma consequent to an accident. The concept of a 'compensation neurosis' that can only be resolved in the personal injury court is unhelpful and unfounded.

Pathophysiology

Acute muscle injury may be the cause of pain in the acute stages. Muscle spasm of the scalene muscles may be responsible for some of the neurological symptoms referred to the arms, including a functional thoracic outlet syndrome. Damage to the recurrent laryngeal nerve may explain other symptoms, such as hoarseness. Primary brain injury may also occur, and be responsible for a psychological disturbance in the chronic syndrome. Significant injuries that can be observed post mortem in victims of lethal trauma include cervical spine fracture and prevertebral haematoma.

It is claimed, on the basis that local anaesthetic block of the nerve to the cervical zygapophyseal (facet joints) temporarily relieves the pain in approximately 50% of patients, that these joints are the principal origin of the pain. It is further claimed that long-term pain relief and reversal of psychosocial morbidity can be achieved by destruction of these nerves. The assumption from this research is that neck pain typically (but not exclusively) associated with rear-end impact is due to an arthritic process in the cervical facet joint.

Other mechanisms which have been suggested to be of importance in the symptom complex include:

- Damage to the sympathetic autonomic supply to the head.
- The cilio-spinal reflex (neck pain associated with ipsilateral pupillary dilatation).
- Altered proprioceptive information from abnormally active cervical efferents leading to disordered vestibular function.
- Reflex inhibition of muscles supplied by segmental levels which receive nociceptive inputs.

Such mechanisms may lead to diverse, sporadic and unpredictable symptoms that may be inappropriately and erroneously attributed to psychological mechanisms:

- Visual disturbance.
- Vestibular difficulties.
- Weakness and heaviness of the arms.
- Paraesthesiae of medial side of hand.
- Dysphagia/hoarseness.
- Auditory disturbance.

Investigation

No investigation is needed to confirm the clinical diagnosis of whiplash injury, but the circumstances of the injury usually require that a lateral X-ray of the cervical spine is taken. Fractures of the cervical spine can occur without impact, and specialized views, e.g. laminar and pedicle views with computed tomography (CT) examination, may be needed.

Treatment

There are many techniques used for the treatment of acute symptoms following whiplash injury. Their efficacy has been critically reviewed. With the exception of mobilization and exercise, which have been shown to provide a short-term benefit, none of the physiotherapy techniques traditionally used for musculoskeletal pain have been proven to be valuable. Indeed, some treatments, such as prolonged rest and the use of a cervical collar, are associated with a worse long-term outlook.

The concept of the pain syndrome being explained in its entirety by an arthritic process secondary to damage to the apophyseal joints is an attractive hypothesis, but one which in practice works for only a proportion of patients. Radiofrequency lesioning of the medial branch of the posterior primary ramus may provide long-term pain relief and even resolution of associated symptoms, but the proximity of the vertebral artery to the target nerve is a potential source of serious neurological morbidity if the therapeutic lesion is not accurately controlled and thermocoagulation or spasm of the artery occurs. Other nerve block techniques which have been described include cervical epidural injections, occipital nerve blocks and sympathetic system blocks.

The 'arthritic' hypothesis, while helpful in defining a treatment that is valuable for a proportion of patients, may be unhelpful in rehabilitation of others. There is a danger of attributing a complex and poorly understood collection of symptoms to a single disease process. This danger is that patient and therapist will be 'held up' by a belief that the spine has been damaged. Useful though it may be in providing an effective treatment for some, the idea that a single pathological process is responsible fails to explain the contribution of fear of movement or understanding of causation that stand in the way of musculoskeletal rehabilitation. Patients who believe that they have badly damaged their necks will behave and complain as if they have. Successful management of the chronic pain associated with such a condition involves changing perceptions and beliefs and encouraging movement and activity.

The 'adversarial' system by which redress for injury is sought through the courts is a stressful process in which the honesty of the claimant is challenged, and is hardly likely to encourage the patient to ignore symptoms that frighten or for which inappropriate explanation has been given. Psychosocial distress commonly accompanies many painful conditions. The manifestation of this distress is contingent on factors such as the way in which society treats victims of accidents, the attitude of employers and the benefits system. Thus patients with neck pain following injury may demonstrate illness behaviour in the same way as patients with other painful conditions, and measures to deal with the behaviour may be part of the treatment. It should not mean that the diagnosis of psychosocial distress should prejudice the outcome of legal proceedings.

Cervical spondylosis

Pathophysiology

This diagnosis describes the changes caused by narrowing of the cervical nerve root foramina by bone or cartilage from osteophytes and hypertrophic facet joints. Such a definition supposes that the nerves in the foramina undergo pathological change, and it is to be expected that the sufferer would present with radicular symptoms.

Clinical presentation

The pain syndromes associated with cervical root involvement are well described and consistent, although symptoms in adjacent nerve root territory may compound the clinical picture. Pain in the distribution of the nerve tends not to involve the hand, although paraesthesiae may be experienced. Upper cervical root compression is experienced as pain over the occiput and mastoid area. Nerve root compression is aggravated by axial loading, and by coughing, sneezing, jugular vein compression and extension of the neck.

Investigation

The diagnosis of cervical spondylosis is a radiological one. As with other chronically painful conditions of the spine, there is a poor correlation between the radiological appearance and the symptoms.

Management

The contribution of the cervical facet joints to the overall pain syndrome can be assessed by specific diagnostic nerve blocks (medial branch of dorsal primary ramus) or intra-articular steroid injection. Cervical epidural steroid and paravertebral injections may be used for pain with radicular features. It is noteworthy that there has been a case report of a high tetraplegia following a properly conducted cervical paravertebral steroid injection.

Electromagnetic field therapy has compared well with placebo for the reduction of pain. Otherwise there is a hierarchy of procedures of increasing difficulty using radiofrequency nerve lesioning techniques that can be used for neck pain with and without nerve root involvement. These are described as:

- Facet joint denervation.
- Stellate ganglion lesion.
- Cervical dorsal root ganglion lesion.
- Cervical disc lesion.

The greater occipital nerve, a continuation of the dorsal ramus of the second cervical nerve, can be blocked just lateral to the external occipital protuberance. Many conditions in which neck pain is experienced are more properly described as one of the musculoskeletal syndromes: cervical spondylosis simply being a convenient clinical description of a radiological observation. As with any other painful musculoskeletal condition, the contribution of psychosocial factors, such as those engendering a fear of movement, should be addressed.

Cervical disc disease

As with lumbar disc disease, cervical disc disease may be completely asymptomatic and be found on imaging. It is common for cervical films to show evidence of osteophytes and loss of disc height with increasing age. A combination of disc prolapse and osteophyte formation produces the clinical picture which may be a combination of radicular effects and myelopathy. Disc prolapse, with or without the addition of root compression due to osteophyte, presents as a combination of neck pain and brachialgia. The neck pain may radiate into the interscapular area and also to the occiput. Brachialgia is in the distribution of the appropriate nerve root and may be accompanied by sensory and motor deficits. In 90% of cases the lesion will be at C5/6 or C6/7.

Myelopathy may occur in association with the features described above or in its own right. Typical is the development of a spastic gait; in addition there may be problems with use of the hands indicating that a quadriparesis is present. Another syndrome, usually typical of compression at C3/4, is 'numb clumsy hands'. Not all cases progress and it is estimated that as many as 40% can be managed conservatively.

Diagnosis

Diagnosis is almost universally by magnetic resonance imaging (MRI), which has all but replaced myelography. If there is signal increase in the spinal cord prior to decompression, in cases of myelopathy, the prognosis is poorer for recovery.

Medical treatment

Medical treatment follows the same principles outlined in the discussion above on cervical spondylosis. Disc abnormalities, as demonstrated with MRI, may be associated with other abnormalities. Whereas a surgical assessment is important to rule out progressively disabling disease, many patients with symptomatic cervical discs can be managed with medical means. Cervical epidural steroids and paravertebral steroid injections may be used, and attention to other features such as the facet joints may be valuable.

Surgical treatment

For single-level disease, the approach is from the anterior; there is disagreement as to whether or not fusion should be performed at the time of disc excision. However, if a simple discectomy is performed then fusion will ultimately result though taking a longer time than if a bone graft is used, and with the possibility of a small amount of kyphosis. The traditional approach is by Cloward's procedure or Smith–Robertson in which some of the vertebral body is removed across the disc space. An iliac crest graft is used to 'plug' the defect and aid fusion after the disc and osteophytic compression of the nerve root has been cleared. Relief of brachalgia in 90% of cases is reported. The same procedure is used in cases of myelopathy, though a difficulty arises when multiple levels are involved. Cloward's procedure can be carried out at multiple levels, but increasingly surgeons may perform a trench vertebrectomy, with grafting and plate fixation. If levels are multiple, then historically posterior laminectomy has been the procedure of choice. For myelopathy the goal is to arrest deterioration, though improvement may also occur.

Further reading

Barnsley L, Lord S, Bogduk N. Whiplash injury. Pain 1994; 58: 283–307.
Ferrari R, Russell AS. Epidemiology of whiplash: an international dilemma. Annals of Rheumatic Disease 1999; 58: 1–5.

Systematic reviews

Gross AR, Aker PD, Goldsmith CH, Pelos P. Physical medicine modalities for mechanical neck disorders. The Cochrane Library, Issue 4, 2000.

Related topics of interest

Back pain – injections (p. 28); Musculoskeletal pain syndromes (p. 95); Nerve blocks and therapeutic lesions – general principles (p. 104); Psychosocial assessment (p. 181).

NERVE BLOCKS AND THERAPEUTIC LESIONS – GENERAL PRINCIPLES

Neural blockade involves reversible (regional anaesthesia) or irreversible (neurolytic blocks) interruption of nerve impulses using specific drugs (local anaesthetics, neurolytic agents). The application of regional anaesthesia and neurolytic methods in a nerve or plexus requires well-established indications and implementation of an agreed therapeutic protocol.

Indications for nerve block in pain management

- Clinical anaesthesia.
- Obstetrics.
- Postoperative analgesia.
- Pain therapy in chronic pain.

Neural blockade in chronic pain

Neural blockade in chronic pain is undertaken for diagnostic, prognostic, therapeutic and prophylactic indications or for a combination of these indications.

Diagnostic and prognostic blocks

Diagnostic nerve blocks are used to determine the source of the pain. These blocks allow differentiation of a local from a referred somatic pain source, a visceral from a somatic pain source, a peripheral from a central aetiology and somatic from sympathetic pathways.

Prognostic nerve blocks are used to predict outcome. These blocks help the patient and the physician decide whether to proceed with surgery or nerve destruction procedures. Diagnostic and prognostic blocks require precise localization of nerve to be of value. Inaccurate needle positioning results in over-optimistic interpretation of the results of definitive treatment. There are several problems associated with the interpretation of results:

- A placebo response.
- Local anaesthetic spreads to adjacent nerves.
- The patient responds to the systemic action of local anaesthetic.
- The nerve block includes the sympathetic nerve fibres and the block is not specific.

In an attempt to improve the accuracy of diagnostic and prognostic blocks, various recommendations have been made to overcome these problems. These are:

- Assessment is made by an observer who is unaware of the treatment.
- Pain relief that outlasts the anaesthetic duration may be due to mechanisms not tested by the nerve block.

- The response to a specific sympathetic block should be ascertained first.
- Low volumes of local anaesthetic agent are used.
- The procedure is undertaken on more than one occasion.
- The patient understands the nature and purpose of the block.

Even when diagnostic nerve blocks are performed with attention to the above details, there can be further problems if it is assumed that nerve destruction or surgery will take away the pain:

- Pain relief can be obtained by nerve block in the area of referred pain rather than to the site of pain itself.
- Pain relief in practice may outlast the pharmacological action of local anaesthetic.
- The dorsal horn will respond to nerve destruction by becoming sensitized.

Despite these limitations, diagnostic or prognostic nerve block of a somatic sensory nerve may be of value even if a negative result is obtained:

- It may convince a patient of the futility of nerve destruction or surgery.
- It may indicate to the clinician that a central component to the pain exists.

Therapeutic nerve blocks

Therapeutic nerve blocks are used to treat painful conditions that respond to nerve blocks.

- Therapeutic nerve blocks are appropriate for alleviating acute pain, especially in a self-limiting disorder (e.g. postoperative, post-traumatic or acute visceral pain syndromes).
- As treatment for exacerbation of chronic pain to provide direct localized therapeutic action.

Local anaesthetic can break the 'vicious circle' of chronic pain and lead to much longer therapeutic actions than might be predicted from the pharmacological action of the drug. Once pain and spasm around a joint have been relieved, movement may become possible. Such an action can be demonstrated after local anaesthetic block to nerves that provide sensory fibres to a joint, but whose motor fibres are not essential for movement of the joint. Examples include the use of obturator nerve block for the painful arthritic hip and suprascapular nerve block for the painful shoulder. The effect may be due to several factors:

- The initial movement around a joint stretches the surrounding structures, leading to a return of normal range of movement. Limited movement due to pain may have resulted in capsular shrinkage and tendon shortening.
- Constant nociceptive stimulation from the site of pain leads to sensitization of the spinal cord, a change which may be reversed with a brief block of the nociceptor afferents.
- The patient gains confidence in moving a limb that has been too painful to move.

- Block of the efferent sympathetic fibres may lead to a change in the behaviour of primary afferent nociceptors that are sensitive to the action of locally released noradrenaline. This effect may outlast the effect of afferent blockade.

Successful procedures may be repeated on an occasional basis. The anatomical explanation for referred pain is one of branching of primary afferents and converging of inputs onto a dorsal horn cell. It can be relieved by local anaesthetic to the site of referred pain. The success of this approach is due to block of tonically active nerve impulses which increase excitability of dorsal horn neurones. Some phenomena of referred pain are difficult to explain but may be treated by imaginative use of local anaesthetic. Examples include pain from angina referred to a recent thoracic vertebral fracture, and pain from sinusitis referred to recently filled teeth. Both visceral and musculoskeletal pains can be treated with therapeutic local anaesthetic nerve blocks of areas of referred pain. Visceral pathology may present with symptoms referred to the somatic dermatomes and local anaesthetic block here may be effective as pain relief.

- Local anaesthetic blocks can be supplemented with other substances for the purpose of therapeutic block. This practice includes the use of corticosteroids, for which there are several rationales. Corticosteroids are indicated to treat presumed tissue inflammation and stabilize nerve membranes, preventing development of ectopic discharges. Nerve membrane stabilization reduces the rhythmic firing of spinal motor neurones by causing hyperpolarization of the resting membrane potential.

Therapeutic nerve blocks help the patient to:

- Maintain an ambulatory or outpatient treatment status.
- Maintain participation in a physical therapy or rehabilitation programme.
- Decrease the need for analgesia.
- In some cases, avoid or delay surgical intervention.

Prophylactic nerve blocks

Prophylactic or pre-emptive nerve blocks are used to prevent painful sequelae. The blocks are established before surgery such as amputation of a limb. There are a few clear benefits of this procedure: these include reduction in the amount of general anaesthesia required; reduction in the stress response to surgery; and better pain control in the immediate postoperative period. The idea that this practice prevents the development of pathological pain such as phantom limb pain remains an attractive, but as yet unproven one, as does the idea that pre-emptive analgesia reduces the requirement for postoperative pain relief.

Conduct of neural blockade

For any nerve block a detailed knowledge of the following is essential:

- Anatomy.
- Indications.

- Contraindications.
- Technique of procedure.
- Pharmacology of drugs.
- Effects of the block.
- Side effects.
- Complications.
- Treatment of complications.
- Limitations.
- Outcome.

A clinician who intends to perform therapeutic injections should be competent to diagnose and manage the specific disorder to be treated. It is not satisfactory to perform a nerve block on the instructions of another clinician without such an understanding.

Resuscitation equipment must be available, along with equipment, monitors and medications, to treat adverse events or complications that might occur. Specifically, the inadvertent injection of local anaesthetic into the vascular system can cause circulatory collapse and the inadvertent injection of it into the cerebrospinal fluid can cause coma and hypotension.

Preoperative care

- Explain the procedure: discuss potential effects, side effects, complications and outcome; specific discussion of any therapeutic substance for which there is no licensed indication is required (e.g. epidural steroid).
- Advise the patient on post-procedure care: document the discussion; determine the patient's neurological status – exclude neurological abnormalities; consider contraindications.
- Absolute contraindications are lack of patient consent, allergy to the medications, coagulopathy, local sepsis or septicaemia.
- In cases where patients are taking anticoagulants, a decision has to be made about discontinuing the medication on the understanding that patients with certain conditions, e.g. prosthetic heart valves or following coronary artery stenting, are more at risk if anticoagulants are stopped even for a short period of time. Ideally the risks and benefits of discontinuing the anti-coagulation should be discussed.
- When there is stable systemic neural disease or local nerve damage, a careful assessment of risk–benefit ratio must be made and discussed with the patient.
- Obtain informed consent.
- Ensure optimal positioning of patient.
- Secure intravenous access.
- Decide on how sedation will be given and monitored, if necessary.

The procedure

- Perform an aspiration test before and during the injection.
- Administer test dose where appropriate.
- Inject medications in incremental doses.

- Maintain verbal contact with the patient.
- Observe for side effects or complications.

Maintain a careful record of the procedure, in particular anatomical abnormalities, instrumentation problems, injection pain, blood aspiration, paraesthesia and complications.

Special reference to nerve blocks for chronic pain

- Knowledge of the natural history and expected clinical course of the chronic painful conditions should influence the physician's judgement as to what procedure should be performed, the necessity of the procedure and the likelihood of success, and lead to true informed consent.
- The treating physician should be aware of alternative or accessory therapies that can be applied before or following procedural intervention and which may enhance the efficacy of the treatment.
- The facility to admit patients and the availablity of on-call doctor's advice and care is occasionally needed. Not all patients can be discharged home straight away: transient weakness or numbness of limbs are causes of disability that may make it inadvisable to return home until recovery has taken place.
- Further objective and meaningful information can be obtained using preoperative and postoperative visual analogue scales (VAS), pain and disability scales, quality of life measures and injection specific questionnaires.

Neurolytic or irreversible neural blockade

Neurolytic procedures are available as part of the management option for chronic pain and their use is mainly based on the expertise of the pain specialist and the needs of a select group of patients. There are four mehods of neurolysis:

- Chemical neurolytic blocks.
- Cryoablation.
- Radiofrequency lesion generation.
- Neuroablative procedures.

The major hazards of nerve destruction techniques are:

- Permanent motor block.
- Neuropathic pain as a consequence of dorsal horn sensitization.
- Accidental damage to structures adjacent to the target nerve.

Chemical neurolytic block

The techniques require the administration of an agent that is capable of destroying neural structures and is used to treat severe pain due to cancer and other chronic non-malignant conditions. The agents that are used for chemical neurolysis are phenol, ethyl alcohol, hypertonic saline and other miscellaneous agents.

Phenol (6%) in glycerol is a hyperbaric solution and causes nerve destruction by inducing protein precipitation. It has an immediate local anaesthetic effect due to its immediate selective effect on smaller nerve fibres and causes a warm sensation. Phenol has systemic side effects including central nervous system stimulation, cardiovascular depression, nausea and vomiting. Doses less than 100 mg are less likely to cause serious side effects. For intrathecal phenol blocks, the patient should lie on the side of the lesion as the solution is hyperbaric. An aqueous, isobaric solution is used for lumbar sympathetic blocks and peripheral nerve blocks.

Alcohol. Ethyl alcohol (50–95%) has a similar destructive effect to phenol and is more efficient in destroying nerve cell bodies. It is available as a 95% solution. Local anaesthetic is used as a diluent. Following its injection, the patient complains of severe burning pain along the nerve distribution which may last for a minute and is subsequently replaced by a warm, numb sensation. Alcohol is used in sympathetic and coeliac plexus blocks for inoperable carcinoma of the pancreas or liver. In intrathecal alcohol neurolysis, the patient is positioned with the target root uppermost as absolute alcohol is hypobaric.

Hypertonic saline. 10% aqueous solution is available and the mechanism of neurolysis is not well known. It causes severe pain on injection, and hence local anaesthetic is first injected prior to the saline solution. When administered intrathecally, hypertonic saline can cause an increase in the intracranial pressure and an increase in blood pressure, heart rate and respiratory rate.

Miscellaneous agents. Ammonium salt solutions, chlorocresol and distilled water have been used in the past with varying results.

Complications of chemical neurolysis. Complications comprise tissue necrosis and sloughing, neuritis, anaesthesia dolorosa, prolonged motor paralysis, perineal and sexual dysfunction and bladder and bowel dysfunction. Systemic complications include hypotension secondary to sympathetic block, systemic toxic reactions, heart rate and rhythm disturbances, blood pressure changes, central nervous system excitation and depression.

Cryoablation

Pain relief from destruction of nerves following exposure to extreme cold is called cryoanalgesia. Cryoanalgesia was used in 1938 by Fay and Smith to promote tumour regression. The term cryoanalgesia was coined in 1976. The major advantage of this procedure is the absence of neuritis or neuroma formation and prolonged analgesia with reversible effect. It has no systemic side effects and produces minimal tissue damage. It is performed as an outpatient procedure. The results are variable.

Radiofrequency lesion generation

This is a technique by which high-frequency electrical current (1 MHz or more) delivered via an insulated probe causes heating of adjacent tissue via an ionic effect, the current being dispersed via an earth electrode connected to the patient. The size of the resulting nerve lesion is affected by the dispersal of heat from the surrounding tissues, and, for normally vascularized tissue, is dependent upon the size of the electrode tip and the temperature measured at the tip. A temperature of 45°C is required to cause damage to C fibres. The resulting effect of heat dispersion through local blood flow is one of allowing precise temperature gradients around a probe of given size and tip temperature that is predictable. For normally vascularized tissue, the radius of heat-induced damage to nociceptive fibres is precise and independent of the duration of current. For needles placed into intervertebral discs, the heat dissipation is much less rapid due to the avascularity of the intervertebral disc, and the size of the lesion is dependent on the length of time for which current passes.

Radiofrequency current is used to ablate pain pathways in the trigeminal ganglion, spinal cord, dorsal root entry zone (DREZ), dorsal root ganglion, sympathetic chain, facet joints and peripheral nerves. Fluoroscopic guidance is a requirement for proper needle placement. Complications include neuritis, neuralgia, numbness and paralysis.

Pulsed radiofrequency is a technique in which the current is delivered in pulses separated by intervals in which heat is dispersed. The result is the delivery of current, with ionic effects, but with the temperature of the tissue around the needle tip kept at about 43°C. Reports of long-acting pain relief, presumably consequent on C-fibre inactivation, have been claimed. The mechanism by which pulsed radiofrequency current delivers a nerve lesion effect is uncertain: heat inactivation or heat-mediated destruction of the nociceptor fibres is clearly not involved. This technique may be particularly valuable for producing nerve lesions in target tissue where nociceptor fibres and somatosensory fibres subserving touch exist in close proximity, for example in the dorsal root ganglion and in peripheral neuromata.

Neuroablative procedures

The principle is to interrupt sensory pathways to the brain or in the brain or brain stem. These invasive treatment modalities include neurectomy (cranial neurectomy, peripheral neurectomy, sympathectomy), DREZ lesioning, cordotomy and brain lesioning techniques such as commissurotomy, mesencephalotomy, thalamotomy and cingulotomy. They are dealt with in a separate chapter.

Further reading

Back pain – injections (p. 28); Neurosurgical techniques (p. 161).

NERVE BLOCKS IN CANCER PAIN MANAGEMENT

The use of nerve blocks in cancer is less widespread than it has been. A better understanding of the use of opioids, improvements in preparations of strong opioids, and acceptance that issues around tolerance and addiction can be ignored together with advances in psychological support, have resulted in an improvement in cancer symptom control. Nevertheless it was estimated, in 1989, that 10% of patients treated with morphine and similar drugs could not tolerate treatment, and a further 10% obtained no significant pain relief. Even with the introduction of alternative methods of opioid delivery, such as the spinal route, there remains a group of patients in whom a nerve block or nerve destruction procedure is appropriate. If successful, a total or substantial reduction in opioid dose and associated side effects will be achieved. Nerve destruction is optimally carried out after assessment of the response to a local anaesthetic block: this step may be omitted if urgency or logistics dictates and the indications for nerve destruction are obvious. A local block may be of value, however, in that a response to a block may outlast the pharmacological action of the local anaesthetic, and chemical neurolysis may be postponed while repeat local anaesthetic procedures are carried out.

Indications for nerve blocks

Pain should be localized or unilateral. Many patients with cancer have more than one pain: in this case, the pain site that is considered for nerve block should be considered to be a major problem in its own right. Visceral and somatic pain is more appropriately treated with nerve blocks than neuropathic pain. Opioids should have been tried and found wanting, either because of failure to achieve analgesia or because of unacceptable side effects.

Choice of method

Block of the sympathetic ganglia or chain is effective for the treatment of visceral pain, and has the specific advantage over blocks of the somatic nerve roots of preserving bladder and bowel control and normal sensation and movement. The choice lies between somatic blocks – intrathecal, epidural, peripheral nerves, interpleural – and blocks of the sympathetic ganglia or the nerves travelling through them.

Specific techniques

1. Intrathecal injections. The intrathecal route for neurolysis is particularly useful for unilateral pain that is limited to the distribution of a few dermatomes. Major side effects are sensory and motor loss, and loss of sphincter control. Intrathecal injections of neurolytic substances are used to destroy the dorsal (sensory) root of the spinal cord. The technique depends on the influence of gravity in distributing hypobaric and hyperbaric solutions of neurolytic substances through the cerebrospinal fluid, and the patient must be positioned accordingly. Furthermore, it is important to remember that the spinal cord is shorter than the spinal column and, that for lesions of the lower thoracic roots, lumbar and sacral roots, the substance must be deposited at a more cephalad level than the exit foramen. Absolute alcohol is hypobaric, and the patient must be positioned with the target root uppermost. Phenol 5% in glycerol is a hyperbaric solution which requires the patient to lie on the side of the lesion.

Side effects are prevented by a technique which allows the cooperation of the patient to report untoward motor loss. Alcohol causes pain in the appropriate dermatomal distribution, phenol results in a sensation of warmth. These observations allow the conscious patient's position to be altered slightly if, after injection, the target for the lesion has been missed. The block can be repeated, avoiding the risk of using too great a volume of neurolytic substance at any one time.

2. Epidural injections. A more widespread pain than those treated by intrathecal neurolysis can be treated with epidural neurolysis. The placement of an epidural catheter allows the adequacy of a local anaesthetic block to be evaluated, and allows phenol (in aqueous solution) to be added on an incremental basis, thus minimizing the risk of motor block.

3. Interpleural injections. Relief of the pain of tumour in the pleura and chest wall following the interpleural injection of phenol has been reported. The greater, lesser and least splanchnic nerves can be blocked via the interpleural route, as an alternative to coeliac plexus block.

4. Peripheral nerve injections. Many possible clinical indications exist, for example the use of intercostal phenol to treat the pain of an isolated rib metastasis. An alternative is the use of a catheter technique for local anaesthetic infusions. Chemical neurolysis of a nerve trunk will produce motor block and sensory block: in the context in which it is administered (i.e. terminally ill and bed-bound patients) this may be a small price to pay for comfort.

5. Coeliac plexus block. This remains a useful method for the relief of visceral pain associated with cancer of pancreas and stomach. The sympathetic block, in addition, results in an increase in gastric motility, with reduction in nausea and constipation. Following a successful coeliac plexus block, opioid consumption can be greatly reduced. Tumour may alter the anatomy of the region, making the block technically difficult. Neurolytic coeliac plexus block has been shown to be effective in 90% of patients with pancreatic or visceral cancer pain. The principal side effect, and one which has to be considered, is the small risk of damage to the arterial supply of the spinal cord. In the context of the terminally ill or bed-bound patient this may well be an acceptable risk.

6. Hypogastric plexus block. This has an application for the treatment of pain from pelvic malignancy, although, as above, anatomy may be distorted by tumour.

7. Ganglion impar block. This ganglion is located deep to the coccyx and is a useful target for perineal lesions.

8. *Percutaneous anterolateral cordotomy.* This, probably underused technique, is appropriate for patients with unilateral pain. The technique involves the positioning of a radiofrequency lesioning probe in the spinothalamic tract at the level of the second cervical vertebra on the side opposite to the pain (the spinothalamic tract crosses the midline of the spinal cord just cephalad to the relevant dorsal horn). The procedure is performed with the patient lying supine and conscious, because the response to stimulation of the spinothalamic tract has to be noted. It is thus a major undertaking for the type of patient who could theoretically benefit most from it (chest wall pain from lung cancer or mesothelioma). Lesions of the tract corresponding to the lumbar and sacral dermatomes are easier than those for the cervical dermatomes. Immediate complications include respiratory depression from phrenic nerve damage; late complications include central neuropathic pain.

Systematic review

Carr D, Eisenberg E, Chalmers TC. Neurolytic celiac plexus block for cancer pain – a meta analysis. Proceedings of the 7th World Congress on Pain, Paris. Seattle: IASP Press, 1993; 338.

Related topics of interest

Nerve blocks and therapeutic lesions – general principles (p. 104); Nerve blocks – infusion techniques in chronic pain (p. 114); Nerve blocks – sympathetic system (p. 124); Neurosurgical techniques (p. 161).

NERVE BLOCKS – INFUSION TECHNIQUES IN CHRONIC PAIN

Intrathecal drug infusions are used to control pain in patients suffering from chronic non-malignant pain (CNMP), cancer pain and spasticity and, although some general principles apply, each area is considered separately. The primary motivation is to take advantage of the lower doses that can be used, thus obtaining greater efficacy with fewer side effects; however, the direct application of drug in the vicinity of the dorsal horn allows for a mechanism of action that could never be achieved by systemic administration as the necessary local drug levels cannot otherwise be achieved.

There are several technologies available, each with its own champions:

- *Percutaneous intrathecal catheter attached to an external pump;* this method is for short-term delivery and used to perform trials of the treatment assessing both efficacy and effectiveness.
- *Totally implanted catheter with a subcutaneous injection port and an external infusion device.*
- *A fully implanted fixed rate delivery system* which consists of a reservoir with a percutaneous refill port; the reservoir is emptied by expansion of a gas-filled chamber, which is compressed by the action of refilling the reservoir with drug. The rate is controlled by a fixed outflow resistance; altering the dose requires refilling of the chamber.
- *A fully implanted programmable system* where the rate is controlled by a battery-operated pump. It is much more flexible than the other methods and doses can be changed by percutaneous programming. It is finding increasing application – such flexibility is important if daily variations in drug delivery rate are required or if the condition is progressive. Compared with fixed-rate devices, reservoir capacity is less. The disadvantage is the relatively high cost.

Common to all of the indications are procedure-related complications, including spinal haematoma, infection, neurological deficits, hygromas and post-dural puncture headaches from cerebrospinal fluid (CSF) leaks. Device-related complications include catheter kinking, dislodgement, disconnection and pump failure, incorrect refill or programme error.

Since a rigorous trial process is required and, subsequently, a refill and troubleshooting service must be provided, this therapy can only be delivered by multidisciplinary teams – these will differ in composition according to the indication (see below), but common to all is the ability to deal with the procedure-related complications. The provision of the technique must be adequately resourced to include monitoring and follow up, time for refills, surgical resources for potential complications and education of the 'team', ward staff, primary carers and relatives.

The three indications are spasticity, chronic non-malignant pain and cancer pain.

Spasticity

Baclofen is administered almost exclusively for this indication. It acts by producing muscle relaxation; therefore the effect is achieved at the expense of a reduction in muscle tone. Too great a reduction may result in loss of function for the patient if he/she depends on a level of tone for weight transfers – accordingly, a trial is performed to assess effectiveness of the treatment; efficacy of baclofen in tone reduction can be guaranteed. The use of programmable pumps may allow for differential dose regimens during a 24-h period – for example, a modest increase may be made overnight to facilitate sleeping and reduced during the day to allow increased function.

Specific indications include multiple sclerosis, spinal cord injury and cerebral palsy. For each of these conditions, good evidence exists for relief of pain where this is secondary to increased muscle tone, although it must be remembered that in such cases pain can result from the secondary consequences of fixed deformities. Often a better sitting posture can be obtained that allows for greater mobility with the use of a wheelchair – this may also help in the prevention of pressure sores. Reduction of tone to allow for independent walking – for example, reversal of the 'scissor gait' in cerebral palsy – is more contentious, and this applies to all claims for improvement in function. However since implantation can almost always be justified on the basis of pain reduction, and since anecdotally there are individuals whose function does improve, this issue does not impact on pragmatic clinical decision making provided the trial does not indicate loss of function. Side effects of intrathecal baclofen do occur – mainly headache and nausea – and respiratory failure is a potential consequence of overdose. Some reduction in respiratory function will occur, although this is trivial except in the circumstance of severe multiple sclerosis – here preoperative assessment of respiratory function may be required. These three indications are radically different pathologies, and therefore the multidisciplinary collaborations – which are critical – are with different disciplines. It is not in the scope of this book to explore this in detail other than to stress the importance of such collaborations.

Chronic non-malignant pain

The principal drug used is morphine, commonly in combination with bupivacaine and clonidine. As a simplification, it can therefore be stated that the pain should be opioid-sensitive, but no clear consensus yet exists regarding choice and combination of drug. Care is also necessary in converting a patient from systemic to intrathecal dosage. Here the assessment and trialling of the patient is the most difficult of all the indications. A multidisciplinary pain team must be involved – psychological assessment is considered mandatory by many, including the authors.

There is not as yet clear consensus regarding the indications. However intrathecal drug delivery (ITDD) is most appropriate in patients with uncontrolled bilateral or axial pain, despite adequate trials of systemic drugs. The technique has been shown to be of benefit in failed back syndrome and chronic mechanical back pain. It may be helpful in neuropathic pain of spinal cord origin: the importance of the trial and assessment process is re-emphasized. In this context there is interest in new agents such as ziconatide. A 'competitor' treatment is spinal cord stimulation (SCS): as yet there is no agreement as to when one technique is favoured over the other, but SCS may be favoured if the pain is more focal, and if the efficacy is equivalent by virtue of the fact that the need for regular drug refills is avoided. Cognitive behavioural therapy may be delivered in parallel with ITDD therapy. The importance of long-term commitment of both patient and physician should not be underestimated.

In this context, long-term as well as short-term side effects are important. Perhaps surprisingly, addiction does not seem to be a problem; however, long-term effects of intrathecal morphine include endocrine effects such as weight gain, body oedema, loss of libido, excessive perspiration, hypogonadotrophic hypogonadism and hypocorticism. Catheter tip inflammatory masses have been described, although rare. They can cause neurological impairment and failure of drug delivery. It is thought they may be related to high concentrations of opioids. Bupivacaine can cause motor weakness and haemodynamic instability. Clonidine can cause hypotension, bradycardia and sedation.

Cancer pain

Until recently such techniques have been rarely used in this context, due to the logistics of performing the treatment and the costs of the implanted technology.

It is estimated that about 10% of cancer patients may not achieve satisfactory analgesia with conventional routes of delivery. Some of these patients may be suitable for ITDD. The main indication for using ITDD in cancer patients is failure of conventional routes of administration of analgesics despite escalating dosages with sequential, strong opioids, and/or dose-limiting side effects in those with regional pain, visceral pain or mesothelioma. Spinal analgesia (which includes epidural and intrathecal delivery) is indicated in 3% of cancer patients.

In cancer pain there are reports of improved pain control and fewer complications with the intrathecal route compared with the epidural route.

However there is now good evidence of improved survival in patients with a diagnosis of cancer resulting from improved treatments for the disease itself. A recent randomized controlled trial has demonstrated substantially improved pain control by ITDD compared with best medical management. In addition this trial found improved survival in the ITDD group, and although not a primary outcome measure in the trial, it is, nonetheless, likely to be a genuine effect. The reason for improved survival may be due either to avoidance of sedation in the ITDD group, leading to improved mobility, or to an avoidance of the direct effect of opioids in suppressing the immune response, or to both! All of these factors argue for increased application of this therapy in malignant pain, and that levels of side effects – especially in respect of sedation – previously tolerated from systemic administration of opioid are no longer acceptable.

Assessment must be multidisciplinary – the obvious inclusion is a palliative care team to ensure that best management with systemic treatment has been obtained, but assessment must also include teams appropriate to treat any focal cause for pain such as spinal fixation for metastatic vertebral involvement or radiotherapy or chemotherapy for the disease itself. Consideration should also be given as to whether other interventional pain techniques might be appropriate – for example percutaneous cordotomy.

However this seems to the authors an underused application at present, whose effectiveness is underappreciated and likely to increase.

Miscellaneous

There are some reports of the use of ITDD baclofen for neuropathic pain as a sole agent and also of its use in complex regional pain syndrome (CRPS), where it may be active against the dystonic component of the disease. Finally, trials are in progress to determine if ITDD baclofen may have an adjuvant effect in combination with SCS.

Further reading

Anderson PE, Cohen JI, Everts EC, Bedder MD, Burchiel KJ. Intrathecal narcotics for relief of pain from head and neck cancer. Archives of Otolaryngology – Head and Neck Surgery 1991; 117: 1277–80.

Hassenbusch SJ, Portenoy RK, Cousins M, et al. Polyanalgesic Consensus Conference 2003: an update on the management of pain by intraspinal drug delivery – report of an expert panel. Journal of Pain and Symptom Management 2004; 27(6): 540–63.

Onofrio BM, Yaksh TL. Long-term pain relief produced by intrathecal morphine infusion in 53 patients. Journal of Neurosurgery 1990; 72: 200–9.

Smith TJ, Coyne PJ, Staats PS, et al. An implantable drug delivery system (IDDS) for refractory cancer pain provides sustained pain control, less drug-related toxicity, and possibly better survival compared with comprehensive medical management (CMM). Annals of Oncology 2005;16(5): 825–33.

Ventafridda V, Caraceni A, Sbanotto A. Cancer pain management in cancer pain. Pain Reviews 1996; 3(3): 153–79.

Related topics of interest

Complex regional pain syndromes (p. 60

NERVE BLOCKS – LOCAL ANAESTHETICS

This chapter discusses the pharmacology of local anaesthetics and the way in which they can be used in pain management. It is not intended to discuss specific nerve block techniques used in surgery or after trauma, as a full account of these will be found in textbooks of anaesthesia. The use of local anaesthetic drugs by the oral and intravenous route for the specific treatment of chronic pain conditions is dealt with in a separate chapter.

Local anaesthetic agents cause the reversible depression of nerve conduction to the area that they are applied. The term local anaesthetic usually applies to the amine or amide esters originally derived from cocaine. There are other drugs which have local anaesthetic properties and include:

- Phenothiazines (chlorpromazine).
- Barbiturates.
- Pethidine.
- Anticonvulsants (e.g. phenytoin, carbamazepine).
- Beta-blockers (e.g. propranolol).
- Antiarrhythmic agents (e.g. disopyramide).
- Antihistamines.
- Amitriptyline.
- Ketamine.

Surface cooling, for example with ice or ethyl chloride, can also be used for local anaesthesia, especially for transient procedures such as injections, manipulations and body piercing, etc.

History of local anaesthesia

Cocaine (obtained from leaves of *Erythroxylon coca*) is a naturally occurring alkaloid, originally found in the foothills of the Andes. For centuries the local tribes used cocaine as a stimulant and were also aware of its numbing effect on the tongue.

In 1860 Neimanns purified the alkaloid. Its local anaesthetic effects were subsequently noted by Moreno y Maiz, who was employed by the Peruvian army. Sigmund Freud began utilizing cocaine as a stimulant and a potential alternative for opium in his addicted friends/clients and on himself (thus becoming an addict). In 1884, Carl Koller, a colleague of Freud, used cocaine for eye surgery. Its medicinal use became widespread and the majority of local anaesthetic techniques/nerve blocks used today were actually described in the first quarter of the 20th century.

Pharmacocokinetics, physiochemical properties and mode of action

Most local anaesthetics share certain similar chemical and physiological/pharmacological properties. They are either tertiary amino esters or amides of aromatic acids. The basic formulae consist of an aromatic lipophilic group, an intermediate chain (ester or amine) and a hydrophilic amine group (secondary or tertiary amine group). The broad classification into esters (procaine, cocaine, chloroprocaine and tetracaine) and amide local anaesthetics (lidocaine, bupivacaine (and its isomers), prilocaine, mepivacaine and etidocaine) is based on the intermediate chain.

In general the esters are relatively unstable, are rapidly hydrolysed (plasma cholinesterase) and have a higher incidence of allergic reactions. The amides are more stable in solution, broken down in the liver by amidases and have a much lower hypersensitivity incidence.

The pharmacological activity of local anaesthetics is a function of their lipid solubility, diffusion across tissues, affinity for protein binding, per cent ionization at physiological pH and vasodilating properties.

Local anaesthetic bases are made soluble in water by their formulation as a hydrochloride salt. This formulation is essential for application but their clinical action requires the presence of the base, unionized form. The relationship between base and ionized form is determined according to the Henderson–Hasselbalch equation that governs equilibrium of acids and bases in solution. For purposes of this illustration the local anaesthetic is denoted by the symbol B_A.

After injection, the (hydrochloride) salt of the local anaesthetic dissociates into its free base:

$$B_AHCl + HCO_3^- \rightleftharpoons B_A + H_2CO_3 + Cl^-$$

The proportions of free base liberated is determined by the tissue pH and the dissociation constant pK_a according to the Henderson–Hasselbalch equation:

$$\log \frac{[B_A]}{[B_AH^+]} + pK_a = pH$$

The free base is fat-soluble and diffuses across the neurone membrane. Once inside, further ionization occurs:

$$B_A + H^+ \rightleftharpoons B_AH^+$$

The ionized form enters the sodium channel (from inside the cell) where membrane-associated proteins are modulated, leading to the sodium channel closure and consequent failure of action potential transmission.

There is thus a balance between free base getting into the cell and the need for its cation to actually cause the molecular effect. Lower tissue pH leads to less free base and therefore slower action/effect; e.g. in ischaemia and infection. Adding bicarbonate to the local anaesthetic solution can speed up diffusion across the cell.

Unionized local anaesthetic base can be formulated for clinical use by its formulation as a eutectic mixture. Eutectic mixtures have physical properties that are different from those of the constituent compounds. A eutectic mixture of local anaesthetics (EMLA) is formulated as a colloid paste that can be applied to skin. The unionized and, therefore, lipid soluble nature of the local anaesthetic makes for effective percutaneous penetration.

As well as affecting clinical activity by sodium channel blockade, local anaesthetics may also work via calcium channel and potassium channel blockade. In addition to these mechanisms, local anaesthetics have been observed to reduce axoplasmic flow. The relevance of these mechanisms is unclear.

Vasoconstrictors can prolong local anaesthetic action and enhance speed of onset by reducing systemic absorption. The reduced systemic concentration allows the dose of some local anaesthetics to be increased, though this phenomenon is not observed with bupivacaine.

Small nerve fibres are blocked at lower concentrations than large fibres. Small preganglionic fibres, the B fibres, of the sympathetic system are particularly sensitive. This accounts for the presence of a sympathetic block after epidural and spinal anaesthesia that occurs in advance of, and at a higher level than, somatic sensory block. Such differential block, as it is known, affects the sensory and motor systems to different extents. Thus Aγ fibres of the extrapyramidal motor system, serving the muscle spindles and responsible for the initiation of movement and regulation of motor tone, will be blocked before the Aα fibres of the corticospinal tract, leading to clumsiness and heaviness of the lower limb. Differential sensory block is also described, with pain and temperature sensation (Aδ and C fibres) being lost before touch and pressure (Aβ fibres).

Local anaesthetics are absorbed into the systemic circulation. In some studies, it has been shown that only 1–2% actually enters the axon. The corresponding peak plasma concentrations depend on the absolute dose given, the blood flow through the tissues and the surface area involved. Thus the rate of absorption is maximum for intercostal block, then caudal epidural, paracervical, epidural, brachial plexus, spinal and infiltration. It can be very rapid from mucosal/bronchial and intrapleural administration. Cocaine can lead to local vasoconstriction, thus delaying its own absorption. Similarly vasoconstrictors can speed up and prolong local anaesthetic action by reducing its systemic absorption. This can allow a significant increase in the total dose (except bupivacaine) that can be used.

After absorption, local anaesthetic is distributed initially to the blood-rich organs. Muscle and fat equilibrate more slowly. The lungs can sequester some local anaesthetics (most noticeable with prilocaine), reducing the load to the systemic circulation.

Ester drugs are broken down in the plasma by cholinesterase (thus, they usually have a short terminal half-life) with only a small amount excreted unchanged by the kidney. Cocaine is an exception, with extensive liver metabolism.

The amide drugs are broken down via amidases in the liver. Some of the metabolites have local anaesthetic properties and can also account for some of the systemic side effects.

Prilocaine is more rapidly metabolized in the liver than the other amides. Some kidney and lung metabolism also takes place. One of its principal metabolites is o-toluidine. This can lead to methaemoglobinaemia, and has been noted in patients who have had large therapeutic doses, especially if they are anaemic. Cases have occurred in children with renal failure, who have had daily applications of EMLA.

The molecule of bupivacaine has an asymmetric carbon atom. With this asymmetric carbon as a chiral centre, bupivacaine exhibits chiral isomerism. In the commercial presentation of this local anaesthetic there is a 50:50 proportion: levobupivacaine, L (–) isomer, and dextrobupivacaine D (+) isomer.

There is a preparation of levobupivacaine that contains only the levorotatory (L) isomer. Interest in levobupivacaine arose after several cases of severe cardiotoxicity (including death) were reported where it was shown that the D isomer of bupivacaine had a higher potential for toxicity. Consequently, it is felt that for levobupivacaine the risk for cardiotoxicity is less.

Local anaesthetic toxicity

This occurs with excess levels of local anaesthetic on the heart or central nervous system (CNS). Toxic peak levels occur because of absolute overdose or inappropriate administration/intravascular injection.

CNS toxicity can lead to feelings of light-headedness, dizziness and circumoral paraesthesiae. Visual and/or auditory disturbances such as difficulty focusing, double or blurred vision and tinnitus can occur. The signs of CNS toxicity (often excitatory) include shivering, muscular twitching and tremors initially involving muscles of the face, hands and feet. Generalized grand mal convulsions can follow. Medullary depression with respiratory and autonomic effects can occur if sufficiently high levels are attained. The rate of progression of the above signs and symptoms can be very rapid and unpredictable.

Cardiovascular toxicity usually occurs at blood concentrations greater than those required to effect the CNS. Cocaine increases the heart rate and blood pressure and precipitates dysrrhythmias via central sympathetic nervous system effects and via inhibition of noradrenaline uptake by peripheral nerves.

Most other local anaesthetics have membrane-stabilizing properties and prolong PR and QRS intervals. The general effect on the heart is depressant, with negative chronotropic and inotropic effects. However dysrhythmias can occur via re-entrant mechanisms (especially bupivacaine, which also has cardiac calcium effects). Severe cardiac dysrhythmias such as resistant ventricular fibrillation and *torsades de pointes* may occur.

In general, a direct relationship exists between the anaesthetic potency and cardiovascular depressant potential of local anaesthetics. The more potent drugs including bupivacaine and etidocaine, have been reported to cause rapid and profound cardiovascular depression in some patients following accidental intravascular injection. This is the rationale for their contraindication in intravenous regional anaesthesia (IVRA).

On the peripheral vascular system, cocaine is a vasoconstrictor. The other local anaesthetics have variable, often dose-dependent, effects on vascular tone. Very low doses can increase vascular tone, but with increasing dose, vasodilatation occurs.

Clinical use

1. Topical application. Topical anaesthesia for eye surgery is widely used. Several local anaesthetics exist in topical form for application to the skin: e.g. EMLA (eutectic mixture of local anaesthetic: lidocaine and prilocaine) and tetracaine (Ametop). This produces surface anaesthesia for minor procedures and venepuncture. Mucous membranes such as the urethra and upper respiratory tract can be also anaesthetized via topical local anaesthetics and gels.

In pain management, lidocaine 5%-impregnated patches are available to apply to areas of allodynia that may occur after shingles or with other neuropathic states. These patches also provide a physical barrier on the skin, reducing the pain of mechanical allodynia further.

2. Infiltration. Superficial injection of local anaesthetic which anaesthetizes the nerve terminals (usually quite rapid).

3. Conduction blockade. Application of local anaesthetic to a nerve fibre leading to blockade of all the modalities of that nerve fibre including the sympathetic efferents travelling with the blood vessels. Examples include femoral nerve block, sciatic nerve block and brachial plexus block.

4. Intravenous regional anaesthesia is a technique whereby a limb is isolated by tourniquet and has local anaesthetic injected into the venous system. The anaesthetic is absorbed onto major nerves and more distally onto peripheral nerve terminals via the vasculature. Short-acting surgical procedures can be performed on the limb. Bupivacaine is contraindicated in IVRA.

5. Continual infusion. Almost any local anaesthetic technique can be prolonged by an infusion of the anaesthetic, usually via a catheter, to the site of administration. Long-term implantable infusion pumps exist for subarachnoid infusion, in chronic pain and palliative care.

In some cases, however, repeated administration via any route leads to tachyphylaxis and/or tolerance and reduced efficacy of the local anaesthetic. It seems more common with continual stimuli/pain or hyperalgesic states. Opiate/local anaesthetic combinations seem to have a synergistic reducing effect on tachyphylaxis. This combination is popular for epidural analgesia.

Central neuraxial blockade: the sensitization model and the theory of pre-emptive analgesia

Extradural administration of local anaesthetic blocks the spinal nerves as it traverses the epidural space, leading to variable degrees of analgesia or anaesthesia. Subarachnoid administration of local anaesthetic affects both the spinal nerves and the spinal cord directly, leading again to variable degrees of analgesia or anaesthesia. Both abolish efferent sympathetic activity – the preganglionic myelinated B fibres are exquisitely sensitive to local anaesthetic – but will leave some of the functions of the sympathetic chain intact. Paravertebral block achieves a unilateral blockade of the sympathetic chain and ganglia as well as segmental somatic analgesia and it is thus claimed that this technique uniquely has the potential for protecting the spinal cord from the unwanted effects of afferent nociceptor activation.

In chronic pain states and neuropathic pain, it has been shown that the analgesic action of local anaesthetic outlasts the 'pharmacological' effect. This effect may be due to the delay in the initiation of the long-term neurophysiological changes that occur with continuous nociceptive afferent activation. This observation, and the model that appears to explain it, supports the idea that in other fields of pain relief, for example after surgery, local anaesthetic blockade, whenever it is technically possible and safe, should be part of an anaesthetic technique. The doctrine of 'pre-emptive analgesia' claims that pain relief administered (in this case as local anaesthetic blockade) before surgery will be more effective than that administered after the spinal cord has been sensitized.

Demonstration of the validity of the sensitization model in the acute pain relief of surgery has been very difficult in practice. In terms of clinical studies, only patients subjected to elective surgery for a non-painful condition are suitable candidates for a rigorous examination of the model. Trial design requires that control subjects are allowed to experience the effects of surgery before analgesia is given, and this may be difficult to justify on ethical grounds. The ability of extradural analgesia to provide pre-emptive analgesia has not been proven, but the ability of paravertebral block to provide pain relief for longer than the expected duration of the local anaesthetic is a well-recognized phenomenon that supports the idea that the sensitization process may have been modified.

Further reading

Lonnqvist PA. Pre-emptive analgesia with thoracic paravertebral blockade? British Journal of Anaesthesia 2005; 95: 727–8.

NERVE BLOCKS – SYMPATHETIC SYSTEM

Nerve blocks of the sympathetic nervous system are indicated for the control of pain where nociceptive afferents travel with the nerves of the autonomic system, or where an effect of blockade of the efferent autonomic nervous system is required. Efferent autonomic blockade has two major effects:

- Removal of the influence of catecholamines from nociceptors.
- Increased blood flow.

The analgesic effects of sympathetic block can be usefully considered as direct and indirect effects. Direct effects result from the removal of a nociceptive pathway, and indirect effects from the modulation of the nociceptive pathway, such that it is less sensitive to the effects of stimulation. This mechanism may be of importance in the pathogenesis of 'sympathetically mediated pain'. Catecholamines are implicated in the process of sensitization of primary afferents in nociceptive and neuropathic pain.

The sympathetic nervous system arises from the spinal roots of the thoracic and lumbar segments. Preganglionic fibres exit from the spinal nerve as the white communicating ramus and pass to ganglia on the paravertebral sympathetic chain. Some fibres pass through the ganglion as preganglionic fibres and synapse in more distal ganglia, from which fibres are distributed along blood vessels. Others form synapses within the ganglion, and postsynaptic fibres form the grey communicating ramus which joins the mixed spinal nerve. Visceral afferents are not themselves technically part of the sympathetic nervous system although their fibres pass through the ganglia and can be blocked in these ganglia.

The anatomy of the sympathetic nervous system lends itself to selective nerve blockade, which can be achieved without motor or somatic sensory loss. Local anaesthetic blockade is sometimes performed as a 'diagnostic' procedure, to enable information to be obtained about the influence of the sympathetic system on the pain. Although the short-term results of sympathetic block may be successful in, for example, reducing the pain of a complex regional pain syndrome, the long-term effects of permanent nerve blockade cannot be guaranteed.

Description of sympathetic nerve blocks is given with reference to the major anatomical landmarks of the sympathetic nervous system.

Stellate ganglion

Three cervical sympathetic ganglia are formed from the fibres which originate from the upper thoracic nerve roots. The lowest of these fuses with the first thoracic ganglion to form the stellate ganglion, which lies superficial to the prevertebral fascia overlying the prominent anterior tubercle of the seventh cervical vertebra. An anterior approach, facilitated by retracting the carotid sheath laterally, is possible at this level. Local anaesthetic block results in a block of the sympathetic supply to the cerebral vasculature, the eye and the upper limb, as evidenced by a Horner's syndrome and warmth in the upper limb. Complications include accidental injection into the vertebral artery, the epidural space and the subarachnoid space. These risks require that the procedure is performed where there are facilities for resuscitation. The proximity of the recurrent laryngeal nerve and the cervical nerve roots accounts for the minor inconvenience of block of these nerves.

Thoracic paravertebral chain

Direct approach to the thoracic sympathetic chain is complicated by the close proximity of the pleura to the chain, and the risk of pneumothorax. However, the interpleural technique of nerve block, involving the positioning of a catheter between visceral and parietal pleura, affords one way of achieving block of the thoracic chain and the nerves associated with it, namely the greater, lesser and least splanchnic nerves. An alternative technique, which does not involve the needle being deliberately introduced into the pleural cavity, is the thoracic paravertebral injection. In this technique, somatic and sympathetic fibres are blocked.

Coeliac plexus

The coeliac plexus lies anterior to the aorta and surrounds the coeliac artery. It consists of three paired ganglia in which fibres from the greater, lesser and least splanchnic nerves form synapses, and through which visceral afferent fibres pass. The technique of coeliac plexus block involves the passage of needles, either side of the aorta, at the level of the body of the first lumbar vertebra, using a posterolateral approach. Needles are advanced from a point 6–7 cm from the midline under X-ray control, to a position in front of the first lumbar vertebral body. Several variations of the technique have been described, including a transaortic approach, in which the needle is passed through the aorta, transcrural and a retrocrural approach, and the use of computed tomography imaging to aid needle localization. The most notable complication, and one which limits the application of an effective technique to patients with limited life expectancy, is the development of paraplegia as a result of damage to the arterial supply to the spinal cord. This complication has been variously attributed to direct needle damage, arterial spasm, direct injection of neurolytic solution or spread of neurolytic solution. Side effects of coeliac plexus block have been estimated as follows from pooling of data from several reports: local pain in 72%, diarrhoea in 41% and hypotension in 36%, with the incidence of more serious side effects occurring in 3%.

Lumbar sympathetic chain

The lumbar sympathetic chain can be interrupted where it lies anterolateral to the lumbar vertebral body. In this position it lies conveniently separated from the lumbar plexus by the psoas muscle. The percutaneous approach to the sympathetic chain involves passage of a needle from a position some 7–8 cm lateral to the midline. With this approach, the transverse process may not be encountered. The classical technique sought the transverse process as a landmark and then reintroduced the needle to pass to the anterior aspect of the vertebral body. Using X-ray control, a mandatory requirement, the landmark of the transverse process can be ignored. X-ray contrast should be seen to be dispersed medially when the needle is in the correct position: lateral spread implies injection into or posterior to the psoas muscle, with the risk of damage to the lumbar plexus. The technique of lumbar sympathectomy carries with it a risk of genitofemoral neuritis that seems to be not influenced by the care that is taken to avoid depositing neurolytic solution on the genitofemoral nerve.

Superior hypogastric plexus

The superior hypogastric plexus lies retroperitoneally at the junction of the fifth lumbar vertebra and the sacrum, and is a bilateral structure. The technique of approach is analogous to that of percutaneous block of the lumbar sympathetic chain, except that the needle is advanced caudally to pass between the transverse process of the fifth lumbar vertebra and the sacral ala. This can be very difficult to achieve, particularly as the gap between the two may be very narrow and the fifth lumbar nerve is in close proximity. Successful treatment of a variety of pelvic pain syndromes, including cancer, has been reported.

Peripheral autonomic system

The technique of intravenous regional anaesthesia involves the use of a sympathetic system-blocking drug, such as guanethidine, being administered into a limb that is isolated from the rest of the body by a tourniquet. The tourniquet itself may have an effect on the function of the autonomic system. All local anaesthetic nerve blocks have the ability to block autonomic fibres as well as the somatic sensory and motor fibres.

Clinical indications

Block, either with local anaesthetic or neurolytic solution, of afferent nociceptive fibres is a valuable technique for the treatment of visceral pain arising from structures served by the appropriate ganglia. On the other hand, neurolytic block of efferent fibres is a more controversial subject. Block with local anaesthetic may help establish the role of the sympathetic nervous system in complex regional pain syndromes and neuropathic pain conditions such as post-herpetic neuralgia, and repeated procedures may allow for extensive rehabilitation by offering short-term pain relief at regular intervals. Block of the sympathetic nervous system is useful for the treatment of limb ischaemia and Raynaud's phenomenon.

Further reading

Plancarte R, Amescua C, Patt RB, Aldrete A. Superior hypogastric plexus block for pelvic cancer pain. Anesthesiology 1990; 73: 236–9.

Systematic review

Carr D, Eisenberg E, Chalmers TC. Neurolytic celiac plexus block for cancer pain – a meta analysis. In: Proceedings of the 7th World Congress on Pain, Paris. Seattle: IASP Press, 1993; 338.

Related topics of interest

Complex regional pain syndromes (p. 60); Nerve blocks in cancer pain management (p. 111); Neuralgia – post herpetic (p. 131); Pelvic and vulval pain (p. 168).

NEURALGIA AND PERIPHERAL NEUROPATHY

A neuropathy refers to dysfunction in a nerve secondary to nerve damage. It can affect a single nerve (a mononeuropathy) or many nerves (a polyneuropathy). It may or may not be painful. A bilateral symmetrical neuropathy is usually of systemic cause. A painful mononeuropathy is often referred to as a neuralgia.

Pathophysiology

Localized or systemic damage and disease can cause demyelination of nerves and less frequently axonal degeneration. Consequently there is a barrage of afferent impulses to the dorsal horn of the spinal cord. This results in central sensitization. Ectopic impulse generation occurs both at the sites of damage and from associated degeneration in the dorsal root ganglion and the spinal cord. Damaged axons become hypersensitive to mechanical and chemical stimuli. Different nerves are affected by different types of damage. Damage may be non-selective, may affect only large fibres or may affect only small fibres. The type of fibre affected has bearing on the symptoms. Although the presence of pain is not related to fibre size alone, damage to smaller fibres more often tends to cause pain. Rapid degeneration is more likely to cause painful neuropathy. Ephaptic transmission (neural cross-talk) causes the provocation of pain by normally non-painful stimuli such as touch.

Painful polyneuropathies

Painful polyneuropathies tend to have a systemic cause. They are most frequently due to toxic agents, metabolic disorders or vitamin deficiencies. They present various patterns of sensory, motor or autonomic deficit. The lower limbs are usually affected, with sensory symptoms prevailing over motor symptoms. The more common ones are described below.

Diabetic neuropathy

This is caused by small-fibre damage. Sensorimotor deficiency and autonomic instability occur. Pain is tingling, burning, stabbing or shooting. Pain may also be due to peripheral vascular disease, joint disease or the development of ulcers secondary to reduced sensation.

Alcoholic neuropathy

This is compounded by concurrent dietary insufficiencies. Non-selective damage occurs, causing a sensory and motor deficit. Pain is burning, with tenderness of the feet and legs.

Nutritional deficiency neuropathy

Vitamin B_1 and niacin deficiencies cause peripheral neuropathy. An associated condition, burning feet syndrome, does not necessarily have the clinical signs of peripheral neuropathy but responds to dietary enhancement of the B vitamins.

Neuropathy due to drugs

Neuropathy from isoniazid therapy is characterized by spontaneous pain and paraesthesiae, worse at night. It is due to large-fibre damage. Other toxic agents include certain chemotherapy agents, arsenic and mercury.

Painful peripheral neuropathies also occur in hypothyroidism, myeloma, amyloid, Fabry's disease, acquired immune deficiency syndrome (AIDS) and as a dominantly inherited form. The peripheral neuropathy of chronic renal failure is often painless but there may be troublesome paraesthesiae or restless legs.

Painful mononeuropathies and neuralgias

Damage to single nerves results from direct trauma, invasion by tumour, past surgery and compression or entrapment.

Examples include carpal tunnel syndrome, cranial, facial and intercostal neuralgias, radicular pain and meralgia paraesthetica (lateral cutaneous nerve of thigh). Within the distribution of the nerve there is pain with associated numbness, hyperpathia or allodynia. Sometimes this presentation, and the associated disability, is more widespread than the distribution of the nerve itself, and is described as a complex regional pain syndrome (type II).

Management

Suspicion of an undiagnosed or undertreated systemic disease warrants investigation and treatment outside the pain clinic. Dietary neuropathies improve with supplements. Myeloma neuropathy can improve with antineoplastic treatments. Similarly entrapment neuropathies may warrant the opinion of a surgeon.

The treatments specifically for pain follow similar principles for both poly- and mononeuropathies and neuralgias. However extensive areas of involvement in the polyneuropathies often make the use of topical treatments impractical.

- *Physiotherapy.* Exercise and use is said to be important to maintain central input from non-nociceptor afferents.
- *Nerve blocks.* A sympathetic component to the pain may be sought. Sympathetically maintained pain is diagnosed as a response to blockade of the sympathetic nervous system, either by block of a ganglion or the intravenous use of guanethidine. The use of such techniques or drugs to maintain analgesia in response to an initial positive response is controversial, and is not well supported by evidence. Nor does the initial success with a local anaesthetic sympathetic block guarantee long-term success with a neurolytic agent. The difficulty in management of neuropathies with these techniques is that the response is variable and unpredictable. In respect of pain that does not respond to sympathetic block, a local anaesthetic somatic block may be of value to reduce the pain in the short term, but somatic block with

a nerve lesioning technique offers no realistic long-term solution: indeed it may result in a deafferentation pain that is worse than prior to treatment. Somatic blocks may however have a place as part of a strategy of encouraging movement about a painful joint affected by the pain, and it is an attractive, though unproven idea, that local anaesthetic blocks allow the central nervous system to restore the normal physiology that existed before sensitization. Somatic block may also be undertaken with a combination of local anaesthetic and steroid – the logic here being to reduce oedema that may be contributing to the condition.

- *Topical treatments.* Systematic review has demonstrated that capsaicin 0.075% cream applied four times daily for 4–8 weeks is effective in the treatment of painful diabetic neuropathy. Other topical treatments include the infiltration of the affected nerve with steroid, glycerol injections or the topical application of local anaesthetic or creams. The application of transcutaneous electrical nerve stimulation (TENS) to stimulate nerves proximal to the areas of damage has been reported to be of value.
- *Antidepressants.* Systematic review has demonstrated the value of tricyclic antidepressants (TCA) for many neuropathic pains. Paroxetine, a selective serotonin reuptake inhibitor (SSRI), has been shown to be effective in painful diabetic neuropathy.
- *Anticonvulsants.* Systematic review has demonstrated that the anticonvulsants gabapentin and pregabalin are effective for trigeminal neuralgia and diabetic neuropathy. There have been five studies of the use of pregabalin in painful diabetic neuropathy; in four studies, pregabalin was statistically effective compared with placebo at doses of 300 mg and 600 mg daily.

Systematic reviews

Collins SL, Moore RA, McQuay HJ, Wiffen P. Antidepressants and anticonvulsants for diabetic neuropathy and post herpetic neuralgia: a quantitative systematic review. Journal of Pain and Symptom Management 2000; 20(6): 449–58.

McQuay H, Carroll D, Jadad AR, Wiffen P, Moore A. Anticonvulsant drugs for management of pain: a systematic review. British Medical Journal 1995; 311: 1047–52.

McQuay HJ, Tramer M, Nye BA, et al. A systematic review of antidepressants in neuropathic pain. Pain 1996; 68: 17–27.

Zhang WY, Li Wan Po A. The effectiveness of topically applied capsaicin. A meta-analysis. European Journal of Clinical Pharmacology 1994; 46: 517–22.

Related topics of interest

NEURALGIA – POST HERPETIC

Post-herpetic neuralgia (PHN) is a chronic pain which can occur following acute herpes zoster infection (shingles). Herpes zoster infection results from reactivation of the varicella zoster virus, dormant in perineural tissues, following a primary chickenpox infection. Acute herpes zoster infection may be painful, although 40% of patients do not report pain. PHN is pain persisting after the pain of the acute infection. The demarcation between pain due to acute infection and the pain of PHN is not defined. Some define pain persisting beyond the crusting of acute infective lesions as PHN; others, pain after specified periods from 4 weeks to 6 months since the eruption of acute infective skin lesions. There is therefore no clear definition of PHN.

Pathophysiology

Acute inflammation and ischaemia during the acute infection cause a necrotizing reaction in the dorsal root, the dorsal root ganglion and the dorsal horn. Large myelinated fibres are more extensively damaged and are reduced in number. This allows increased transmission of nociceptive information at the dorsal horn and thereby pain. The elderly have fewer large myelinated fibres. Further reduction in number by disease process explains the susceptibility of the elderly to the development of PHN. Usually only a single dermatomal segment is affected. Damage occurs to both sensory and motor nerves but the effect on motor nerves is subclinical.

Clinical features

If PHN is defined as pain persisting at 1 month, the incidence varies from 9% to 14%. It has been found to be only 3% at 1 year and tends to gradually improve and eventually remit. More severe pain lasts longer. PHN develops almost exclusively in people over the age of 50. It occurs in up to 65% of those over the age of 60. Acute herpes zoster causes pain in a dermatomal distribution. The pain of PHN is in the dermatomal distribution of the acute infection. The commonest sites for PHN are thoracic dermatomes and the ophthalmic division of the trigeminal nerve. It is less common with lumbar dermatomal involvement. It is usually unilateral.

Pain is a constant aching, burning or itching. There are paroxysms of severe stabbing or lancinating pain. Allodynia, hyperalgesia and hyperaesthesia often occur. There is scarring and pigmentation in the affected dermatomal distribution with a wider area of sensory change.

It is now clear that the various manifestations of PHN are the consequence of varying degrees of sensory nerve damage. Thus three 'subtypes' have been described, and distinguished both by clinical features and the response to treatment:

- Irritable nociceptor subtype: damaged primary afferent nociceptors are responsible for the allodynia. There is an exaggerated response to capsaicin and adrenaline infiltration. There is little deficit in sensory thresholds, since sensory signalling still takes place.
- Deafferented allodynic subtype: primary afferents are more extensively damaged. C fibres develop neuromata, which discharge spontaneously. This leads to central sensitization of the dorsal horn. There is a selective loss of C fibres, so sensation to touch is preserved. However, the normal discharges of the surviving Aβ fibres cause the sensitized spinal cord to signal pain when stimulated by light touch.
- Deafferented non-allodynic subtype: the nerve damage is very extensive, the skin is insensitive to all modalities and the pain is a consequence of central sensitization and neuronal reorganization.

Pain can be severe enough to cause lethargy, anorexia, sleep disturbance, loss of libido and consideration of suicide.

Management

Prevention. Currently there is no proven useful therapy for the prevention of PHN. The benefits of aciclovir and corticosteroids require further evaluation. Therefore vigorous efforts must be made to prevent acute herpes zoster infection by vaccination programmes, etc. Opinion is divided as to the role of nerve blocks. Amitriptyline has been suggested as a prophylactic drug.

Treatment

Tricyclic antidepressants. Systematic review of tricyclic antidepressants has concluded a benefit for the treatment of PHN, with a number needed to treat (NNT) quoted as 2.3 for 50% pain relief at 3–6 weeks. Several drugs of the same category may need to be tried. Amitriptyline is recommended at an initial dose of 10 mg nocte in the over-65 age group and at 25 mg at night for those under 65.

Capsaicin. The combined NNT from two trials of capsaicin 0.075% has been calculated to be 5.3. The use of capsaicin, however, is inappropriate in the presence of 'irritable nociceptor' PHN.

Anticonvulsants. There have been four randomized double-blind placebo-controlled studies of the use of pregabalin in post-herpetic neuralgia. Pregabalin was effective in relieving neuropathic pain in three out of the four studies. At 150, 300 and 600 mg daily, compared with placebo, it was statistically significant in relieving pain. The NNT for decreases in pain scores of >30% was 2.7 and for decreases of >50% was 3.4. Gabapentin has been shown to reduce the pain of PHN. Reports of efficacy of carbamazepine and phenytoin have also been made.

Opioids. There is some evidence to support partial effectiveness of opioid drugs in PHN. Morphine has been shown to significantly relieve PHN and results are favourable for another strong opioid agonist, oxycodone.

Local anaesthetic. The application of a 5% lidocaine patch for 12 out of 24 hours for a period of 6 weeks has been shown to be effective in the treatment of post-herpetic neuralgia. Daily subcutaneous injections of local anaesthetic have been reported. This technique may be particularly appropriate for the 'irritable nociceptor' subtype of PHN. Repeated somatic nerve blocks and sympathetic blocks have also been reported. The rationale is the alteration of central sensitivity by the reduction of nociceptive and peripheral neuropathic input into the dorsal horn.

Steroids. Steroids are claimed to be effective both in painful peripheral lesions, and around the nerve root, where reduction of inflammatory processes may prevent neuronal damage.

Transcutaneous electrical nerve stimulation. The benefit of TENS is dependent on there being sufficient innervation from normally conducting fast fibres. In practice, TENS is poorly tolerated where there is extensive allodynia.

Further reading

Rowbotham M, Harden N, Stacey B. Gabapentin for the treatment of postherpetic neuralgia: a randomized controlled trial. Journal of the American Medical Association 1998; 280: 1837–42.
Rowbotham MC, Pertersen KL, Fields HL. Is post herpetic neuralgia more than one disorder? IASP Newsletter, Fall, 1999; IASP Press, Seattle.

Systematic reviews

Lancaster T, Silagy C, Gray S. Primary care management of acute herpes zoster: systematic review of evidence from randomized controlled trials. British Journal of General Practice 1995; 45: 39–45.
McQuay HJ, Tramer M, Nye BA, et al. A systematic review of antidepressants in neuropathic pain. Pain 1996; 68: 217–27.
Schmader KE, Studenski S. Are current therapies useful for the prevention of postherpetic neuralgia? A critical analysis of the literature. Journal of General Internal Medicine 1989; 4(2): 83–9.
Volmink J, Lancaster T, Gray S, Silagy C. Treatments for postherpetic neuralgia: a systematic review of randomized control trials. Family Practice 1996; 13(1): 84–91.
Zhang WY, Li Wan Po A. The effectiveness of topically applied capsaicin. A meta-analysis. European Journal of Clinical Pharmacology 1994; 46: 517–22.

Related topics of interest

Anatomy and physiology (p. 5); Neuromodulation – TENS, acupuncture and laser photo-biomodulation (p. 146); Therapy – antidepressants (p. 209); Therapy – capsaicin (p. 219).

NEURALGIA – TRIGEMINAL AND GLOSSOPHARYNGEAL

There are now recognized a number of neurovascular compression syndromes of which trigeminal neuralgia (TGN) is the best understood. Since this is the one most relevant to a pain practice it is discussed in more detail; of the other conditions glossopharyngeal neuralgia is worth mentioning.

Trigeminal neuralgia

This is an unusual example of a neuropathic pain that may be amenable to surgical correction in which a potential cause is removed.

Incidence and prevalence

The incidence is estimated to be 50/million/year and the prevalence at 155/100 000. It is of increasing frequency with age.

Pathophysiology

In approximately 90% of cases a vessel, usually an artery, is found in contact with the trigeminal nerve at the root entry zone as it exits the pons. Sometimes this contact may groove the nerve. It is not clear how such contacts cause TGN, but sensory malfunction can be detected in the laboratory, as can abnormalities of the trigeminal somatosensory evoked response. Normalization of neurophysiology and sensation occurs following microvascular decompression (MVD), and the usual outcome from the procedure is instantaneous pain relief. All of these observations argue that the neurovascular contact or compression is important in the causation of the condition. It has also been proposed that spontaneous discharges occur within a hyperexcitable trigeminal ganglion – the equivalent of the dorsal root ganglion in the spine where similar behaviour has been observed following spinal injury. The combination of this factor with the effect of neurovascular contact at the root entry zone, perhaps causing demyelination, or a multiple sclerosis (MS) plaque in the trigeminal system results in the paroxysmal nature of the pain and its intermittent course. A total of 2–4% of cases of MS suffer trigeminal neuralgia whilst 5% of cases of trigeminal neuralgia are in association with MS.

Clinical features

The clinical features of the condition have been defined by both the International Association for the Study of Pain and by the International Headache Society. The pain should be unilateral in the distribution of one or more branches of the trigeminal nerve. The pain is sharp and stabbing in quality, coming in paroxysms. There are trigger points which are usually circumoral;

hence the pain is provoked by chewing, talking and wind on the face. The pain is intermittent in nature, with remissions lasting several weeks or months. A response to treatment with carbamazepine is typical and it is refractory to conventional analgesics including anti-inflammatory agents and opioids. In the majority of cases the pain involves the second or third divisions, and only relatively rarely is the pain purely in the first division.

Signs

In classical teaching there are no signs, though a decreased corneal reflex may occur. Therefore any neurological deficit found on bedside testing should raise the suspicion of a structural lesion, or of idiopathic trigeminal neuropathy. However, quantitative sensory testing carried out in laboratory conditions will reveal subtle sensory deficits undetectable clinically.

Differential diagnosis

From a spectrum of other facial pain and headache syndromes, conditions referred for clarification of diagnosis include atypical facial pain, cluster headache, painful trigeminal neuropathy and temporomandibular joint dysfunction. Perhaps surprisingly dental pain is rarely seen in the pain clinic, though a large number of patients have first passed through a dental practice. Although classically described as trigeminal neuralgia, pain from structural lesions such as the extremely rare trigeminal schwannoma or lesions in the region of the cavernous sinus are different, being continuous, progressive and associated with neurological deficit.

Investigations

No specific test exists for this condition. However magnetic resonance imaging (MRI) techniques are now available which detect the presence or absence of neurovascular contact at the root entry zone with a sensitivity of 100% and specificity of 96% validated in a series of 55 cases. The same studies reveal that neurovascular contact may be found in almost 10% of controls so the MRI findings should not be relied on to prove the diagnosis but used to influence the choice of treatment. Some attempts have been made to demonstrate preoperatively neurophysiological abnormalities, particularly far-field evoked potentials, but these have not proven to be either sufficiently sensitive or specific.

Management

The natural history of the condition is for the severity of attacks to worsen and for the periods of remission to shorten. Symptomatically the syndrome may evolve from its typical form to a variant in which there is a constant background burning element to the pain, in addition to the classical features. This variant is termed atypical trigeminal neuralgia. There may also be the development of subtle sensory impairment – in effect the development of a trigeminal neuropathy.

Drug management. The drug of first choice is carbamazepine. Whilst effective, treatment with this drug is not without problems. It is difficult to estimate accurately the numbers of patients who 'fail' medical treatment. Reasons for failure are idiosyncratic reactions to carbamazepine (rash being typical) and dose-related problems. At high dose – to which the patient is driven by the severity of the pain – there may be ataxia and severe drowsiness. However the cognitive impairment produced by the drug 'in normal usage' is underestimated and may be the principal reason why some sources have found failure rates with carbamazepine reaching 75% of cases treated. Analysis of studies concludes that the number needed to treat (NNT) for effective pain relief (>50% compared with control) is 2.6 and the number needed to harm (NNH) is 3.4. One long-term study exists where either loss of effect or intolerance occurred in >50% of patients over 10 years.

Alternatives that have been reported to be effective include lamotrigine, phenytoin, sodium valproate, gabapentin and baclofen. All have been reported to be effective in combination, though there is no published study comparing monotherapy and polytherapy.

Withdrawal of medication should be gradual because of the risk of provoking a seizure; however, although this can occur, it is rare. Patients often stop their medication quite rapidly of their own volition when entering a period of remission without experiencing this complication.

Sodium valproate and phenytoin find application in the acute situation as they can be given intravenously.

Peripheral lesions of the divisions of the trigeminal nerve using alcohol or nerve avulsion. These will not be discussed in detail: save to say that there is a high rate of pain recurrence and late deafferentation pain and cannot be recommended.

Foramen ovale or Gasserian ganglion methods of nerve block. The trigeminal ganglion is approached via the foramen ovale. Fluoroscopic imaging is required.

- *Radiofrequency lesioning.* A needle is introduced via the foramen ovale; electrical stimulation is performed to confirm correct placement of the needle by inducing paraesthesiae in that area of the face where the trigeminal neuralgia is occurring. The patient is then anaesthetized and a thermocoagulation performed (60–90°C for approximately 45 seconds). Although originally suggested that heat preferentially destroyed selectively thin pain fibres, using formal sensory testing it was found that all fibres are affected approximately equally. It is difficult to target the ophthalmic division, and this runs the risk of corneal anaesthesia. A further risk is of masseter weakness and for this reason the technique is rarely performed bilaterally.

  Over 90% will experience immediate relief of pain; however with time there is a gradual recurrence rate. Recurrence rates vary with series, and range from as poor as 25% pain free at 2 years to up to 80% pain free, and the recurrence rate seems to be related to the technique. If deep hypoalgesia is produced during the procedure, essentially by creating a larger lesion, the recurrence rate is lower. Unfortunately the larger the lesion the greater the risk of creating dysaesthesias, and the feared complication of *anaesthesia dolorosa*. In series with low pain recurrence rates, the higher dysaesthesia rate is found; 25% of cases exhibit dysaesthesia regarded by the patient as unpleasant but tolerable. However in 8% treatment is instituted and quality of life assessment indicates that although pain control has been achieved overall quality of life is unchanged. In 1% there is severe disabling *anaesthesia dolorosa*. It will be seen that this complication is only apparent in patients without recurrence, though we have seen it 'revealed' in patients undergoing MVD with recurrent TGN after radiofrequency lesioning.

The procedure is regarded as safe, but is not completely without risk. It involves intermittent anaesthesia in an elderly patient; meningitis and caroticocavernous fistulae are amongst reported complications.

- *Glycerol.* A needle is again placed into the foramen ovale and then glycerol introduced under fluoroscopic control. Accurate positioning of the needle is important. The technique has caused much controversy. In the hands of its proponents excellent results are obtained (best reports being 90% pain free at 1 year); however others report poor results (only 17% pain free at 5 years at worst) with significant dysaesthesia rates, the latter reaching 44% in some series.
- *Balloon microcompression.* The procedure is performed under general anaesthesia. A Fogarty catheter is passed into Meckel's cavity and inflated for between 1 and 6 min. The method has been used since the 1950s. Sensory impairment is produced though mild. The best reported results indicate recurrence of around one-third of cases, though many reports have a much lower success rate, with a dysaesthesia rate of around 10%.

Surgical management

Microvascular decompression of the trigeminal nerve. MVD for trigeminal neuralgia was first carried out by Dandy in the 1930s though the operation was popularized by Jannetta more recently (1967).

Fitness for surgery. Fitness for surgery has been a major issue in the past, particularly in view of the age range with which this condition is often associated. With modern anaesthesia very few patients are unsuitable for this procedure, and the choice between percutaneous radiofrequency lesioning and MVD can be based on the outcomes of the procedures. Series of elderly patients exist in which there is little difference in outcome or morbidity comparing the over-75 age group to those younger. It is worth remembering that radiofrequency lesioning also involves anaesthesia and that this is intermittent.

Operation. This is performed via a retromastoid craniectomy; the subsequent approach is over the surface of the cerebellum until the nerve is identified. Arteries must be dissected free and held clear from the nerve using a small piece of Ivalon sponge or Teflon; if a vein is the cause it may be coagulated and divided. If no vessel is found a partial sensory rhizotomy gives good relief, and, being a centrally placed lesion, appears less likely to give rise to anaesthesia dolorosa; however this procedure is now rarely performed, and not at all in the author's practice.

Risks. In most published series the serious morbidity (death or major stroke) is significantly below 1%. The operation, being performed near to the acoustic nerve, also carries a risk of hearing impairment, possibly due to traction on the nerve whilst retracting structures to gain access to the deeper trigeminal nerve. Since brain stem auditory evoked responses have been used as a monitoring device peroperatively, the risk of unintentional hearing deficit has been reduced to about 2–3% from historical series where risks might be as high as 13%.

Outcomes. Overall, of those with clear arterial compression, a good long-term result will be obtained in about 90%, of whom some 70% are completely pain free up to 20 years postoperatively. Results of venous compression are less good as are the outcomes following partial rhizotomy – approximately 60–70% at 2-year follow up. Case selection is important as poor outcomes from MVD are found in patients with atypical pain or in whom the diagnosis is not TGN. This is why the MRI findings must not be used to confirm the diagnosis – 10% of controls will show contact.

Stereotactic radiosurgery. Some controversy surrounds the results for this technique, in which focused radiation is applied to the root entry zone using the 'gamma knife'. Unfortunately the tendency of units is to report results as 'good' and not specifically stating the true 'pain-free' outcome rate used in other techniques. When this stricter criterion is used, the results are less impressive; the best results find only 65% of patients experience pain relief by 6 months, rising to 75% at 33 months. From this it will be seen that the effect is not immediate; furthermore, only 56% of those who obtained relief also had complete or partial relief at 5 years follow up, implying a high recurrence rate. Finally it has also been demonstrated that there is a dysaesthesia rate; also a dose-related post-radiation numbness.

Choice of technique. The author considers MVD to be the treatment of choice in most instances of severe trigeminal neuralgia whilst recognizing that others may consider that it is a treatment best reserved for failed medical management or may prefer percutaneous nerve lesion technique. MVD corrects a structural abnormality and allows neurophysiological function to return to normal. In all other methods, such as radiofrequency lesion techniques, long-term nerve damage is sustained. These points summarize the reasoning:

- The natural history is for the condition to worsen.
- The side effects of medical management, particularly cognitive, are significant and many patients fail this treatment.
- All destructive lesions (peripheral, foramen ovale, radiosurgery) are associated with a significant recurrence rate: incidence of sensory deficit and production of unpleasant dysaesthetic symptoms or even anaesthesia dolorosa.
- MVD is demonstrated to be effective and of low risk even in the elderly population.
- MRI can detect neurovascular compression preoperatively so that patients with arterial compression can be advised of the likelihood of an excellent

outcome, and patients can be offered an alternative technique if the scan is negative.
- MVD has the best efficacy when published results from all techniques are compared.

Although some good outcomes have been seen following radiofrequency lesioning, more than one series reports that 25–50% only are pain free at 2 years in contrast to MVD where 60–70% pain-free outcomes at 20 years are reported. Over a shorter time period, 44% of patients were pain free at 2 years following balloon microcompression, while similar figures for radiofrequency lesioning were 58% and 75% for MVD. Recent evidence suggests that MVD is followed by normalization of trigeminal somatosensory physiology and cutaneous sensation; thus while trauma to the nerve can be effective (for example, partial rhizotomy), MVD itself should be regarded as a non-destructive procedure for pain relief.

Trigeminal neuralgia as an emergency

Occasionally patients present as an emergency with pain. The patient is drowsy and ataxic, having by this point taken so much carbamazepine as to suffer severe toxic effects, and is furthermore dehydrated being unable to swallow fluids owing to this action triggering the neuralgia.

Management requires admission and bed rest for the ataxia, intravenous fluids to correct dehydration and finally measures to treat the pain. An intravenous loading dose of either phenytoin or sodium valproate is usually effective in treating the pain. This may be followed by emergency MVD or, if MRI is negative for compression, one of the foramen ovale methods.

Glossopharyngeal neuralgia

In reality the anatomy of the lower cranial nerves is such that the glossopharyngeal nerve may be considered as the upper part of a complex which includes itself, the vagus and the cranial part of the accessory nerve.

The syndrome may be considered as identical to trigeminal neuralgia, except in two or three aspects: first, it is considerably rarer; secondly, the distribution of the pain is in the area of the glossopharyngeal nerve. Thus the shooting pain is more within the throat, and triggering is also from the back of the throat. Treatment is identical: the first-line drug is carbamazepine, and surgical decompression provides much the same results as for trigeminal neuralgia. There is no equivalent of radiofrequency lesioning in this condition.

VII/VIII complex

Hemifacial spasm, tinnitus and nervus intermedius neuralgia arise from this complex. MVD is effective for hemifacial spasm, which is the most common manifestation of compression at this level. The procedure for tinnitus is rarely performed and controversial, whereas pure nervus intermedius neuralgia is extremely rare. It can present with otalgia or throat pain. When the predominant pain is in the ear canal, it has been termed geniculate neuralgia.

Further reading

Barker FG 2nd, Jannetta PJ, Bissonette DJ, Larkins MV, Jho HD. The long-term outcome of microvascular decompression for trigeminal neuralgia. New England Journal of Medicine 1996; 334: 1077–83.

Meaney JF, Eldridge PR, Dunn LT, et al. Demonstration of neurovascular compression in trigeminal neuralgia with magnetic resonance imaging. Journal of Neurosurgery 1995; 83: 799–805.

Nurmikko TJ, Eldridge PR. Trigeminal neuralgia – pathophysiology, diagnosis and current treatment. British Journal of Anaesthesia 2001; 87: 117–32.

Tronnier VM, Rasche D, Hamer J, et al. Treatment of idiopathic trigeminal neuralgia: comparison of long-term outcome after radiofrequency rhizotomy and microvascular decompression. Neurosurgery 2001; 48: 1261–68.

Zakrzewska JM, Lopez BC. Trigeminal neuralgia. Clinical Evidence 2004; 12: 1880–90.

Related topics of interest

Facial pain (p. 73); Headache (p. 79); Nerve blocks and therapeutic lesions – general principles (p. 104); Therapy – anticonvulsants (p. 207).

NEUROMATA, SCARS AND CHRONIC POST-SURGICAL PAIN

Chronic pain after surgery is an important and underestimated cause of morbidity. There are several potential causes, and they are discussed here. Nociceptive and neuropathic mechanisms may be involved. An understanding of the nature of chronic pain is important in managing the condition.

Neuromata

Neuropathic pain is pain caused by a primary lesion or dysfunction within the nervous system. The neuroma is the animal model for neuropathic pain. In humans neuromata can cause pain. Neuromata develop following partial transection of a nerve. The initial pain is from A and C fibres firing. An increase in neuronal excitability causing spontaneous discharge of action potential can occur following nerve transection. Ongoing pain, accompanied by allodynia, hyperalgesia and hyperpathia, then occurs.

Pathophysiology

- When a nerve axon is cut the part which is still attached to the cell body forms a swelling (end bulb). Elongating processes are sprouted from the end bulb as an attempt to regenerate. Regeneration occurs if the axonal sprouts reach their target peripheral receptors and normal function is restored. If the processes do not reach their target, sprouting continues and when their forward progress is blocked sprouts become entangled to form a neuroma. Sprouts cause disruption of the myelin sheath. Secondary reorganization of membrane electrical properties takes place, causing neuronal hyperexcitability. This may be due to an increase in number of sodium channels in the proximal axonal membrane.
- Disruption of the myelin sheath produces ectopic foci of electrical activity locally and in sites remote from the damage such as the dorsal root ganglion.
- In undamaged nerves individual afferent fibres conduct independently, insulated by myelin. Where demyelination has occurred, nerves cross-excite each other electrically. This is termed as ephaptic transmission or neuronal cross-talk. When nociceptive afferents cross-excite each other, amplification of pain occurs. However, coupled fibres can be of different types; nociceptor afferents may be activated by afferents for light touch such that allodynia occurs. Ephaptic transmission occurs between afferents and efferents.
- Neuromata are chemically sensitive, for example, to adrenaline and noradrenaline.
- Neuromata discharge abnormally into the central nervous system (CNS) from the periphery. This may cause a phenomenon of central sensitization.

Clinical features

Neuromata are present in sites where the perineurium has been breached but not at all sites where nerves have been cut. Pain from neuromata is variable and may be governed, amongst other things, by genetic factors. Neuromata are often, but not necessarily, palpable as discrete tender lumps. Several neuromata can be found, trapped at a suture line because the regenerating nerve fibres are unable to sprout across them.

- Pain is most intense during the first 2 weeks of the neuroma's development, continuing beyond then but less sustained.
- Pain from the neuroma may be spontaneous or provoked. Pressure on the neuroma may provoke pain through contiguous areas.
- Pain is augmented by percussion of the neuroma. The neuromata may demonstrate allodynia, hyperalgesia or hyperpathia.
- Temperature, metabolic and chemical factors can excite ectopic discharge in animal models.

Treatments

- Systemic administration of drugs acting on the sodium channel can prevent electrical firing. First-line treatment is with anticonvulsants. Local anaesthetics and antiarrhythmics are also used.
- Calcium channel blockers may also have a role in reducing excitability but have not yet been clinically evaluated.
- Surgical excision of neuromata can be effective but in susceptible individuals neuromata recur.
- Mechanically sensitive neuromata can be surgically embedded in deep tissue and in bone marrow away from factors which may encourage nerve growth factor (NGF) production.
- Injections of local anaesthetic into neuromata can have effects outlasting the pharmacological duration of the local anaesthetic.
- In animal models, electrical discharge from neuromata can be decreased by noradrenaline depletion with agents such as guanethidine or bretylium.
- Topical steroids and topical glycerol suppress ectopic neural discharge in experimental neuromata.

Scar pain

Hypertrophic scars regress with time. Gross keloid scars may be suitable for excision. Excision is however almost always followed by a recurrence. Steroid creams and pressure on scars have been used to prevent recurrence. Steroid injections may be more effective. Revision of painful scars is not always successful in producing pain relief and should be undertaken with reservation. It is suggested, but not proven, that prevention of secondary CNS changes by local anaesthetic block can result in less pain after surgery.

Infiltration of the scar with local anaesthetic and steroid has been reported as effective. Cryotherapy to the scar is effective in isolated scar pain. Benefit from sympathetic nerve blocks suggests that pain may have a sympathetic component. Subsequent treatments are repeated sympathetic nerve blockade and the use of drugs which act on the sympathetic nervous system.

Tricyclic antidepressant drugs, anticonvulsants and membrane-stabilizing agents are all used. Radiofrequency lesioning locally to the scar or to the dorsal root ganglion is another option. Such lesions may be more appropriately made with low-temperature (pulsed) radiofrequency techniques.

Chronic post-surgical pain

This refers to pain in and around the operation site. It is a new pain following surgery not a pain which has failed to have been cured by surgery. It may or may not involve the scar, a neuroma or specific nerve damage. It is more likely after the following surgical procedures:

- Thoracotomy.
- Coronary artery bypass grafting, especially after internal mammary artery grafting.
- Sternotomy.
- Breast surgery.
- Inguinal hernia repair.
- Radical neck dissection.
- Cholecystectomy.
- Nephrectomy via flank incision.
- Pelvic surgery via Pfannenstiel incision.
- Episiotomy.
- Strip of the long saphenous vein.

Thoracotomy

It is estimated 50% of patients have chronic pain 2 years after thoracotomy. Recurrent malignant disease must be excluded. Thoracoscopy also causes significant long-term morbidity. Pain may be non-specific neuropathic pain but can be an identified single-nerve neuralgia.

Pain following cardiac surgery

There is a recognized post-coronary artery bypass graft (CABG) pain syndrome. This has been reported as having an overall incidence of 56%. It has clinical features of a neuropathic pain. Pain can also be experienced as a consequence of the sternotomy and the use of the internal mammary artery for graft reconstruction.

Breast surgery

Studies report varying incidences of chronic pain following breast surgery, usually around 30%. It is sometimes referred to as post-mastectomy pain syndrome, even if there has been no mastectomy but only wide local excision. Surgery can vary from wide local excision to radical reconstructive surgery. There are reports of pain persisting for up to 12 years. It is important to exclude recurrent disease as a cause of pain. Pain may be of different causes and more than one cause may coexist in the same patient. To highlight the cause allows more specifically directed treatment. Further axillary node clearance and radiotherapy may contribute to the pain amalgam. The role of preservation of the intercostobrachial nerve is debated.

Causes of pain after breast surgery

1. Recurrent cancer. Patients should remain under the follow-up care of an oncologist or breast surgeon whilst they have persistent pain.

2. Radiation-induced pain. This can be the result of changes in nerve, fat, connective tissue or bone causing oedema, fibrosis, necrosis and ischaemia, or a radiation-induced brachial plexopathy. The description can give an idea as to whether the pain is likely to be nociceptive or neuropathic. Brachial plexopathy has become less common as radiotherapy techniques have improved. It develops late into disease. It is caused by loss of myelin and ischaemia. It presents as pain in the C5/C6 distribution of the treated side and with wasting and weakness of the small muscles of the hand.

3. Post-mastectomy pain syndrome. Neuromata should be excluded. This is a neuropathic pain syndrome but there may be associated nociceptive pain. There may be a sensation of 'phantom breast'. It presents as pain in the axilla, medial upper arm, anterior chest wall or lateral chest wall. There may be associated paraesthesiae, and allodynia is present in 20% 1 month after surgery.

4. Associated conditions. Associated conditions are frozen shoulder, carpal tunnel syndrome and lymphoedema: the latter tends only to be painful if the limb is grossly swollen and heavy or if there is a cellulitis.

An attempt to diagnose pain is helpful but in reality a symptom-orientated approach is used, dividing pain largely into nociceptive or neuropathic categories.

Management

Many of these pains are neuropathic in origin and logic would dictate that tricyclic antidepressants, anticonvulsants, the use of lidocaine patches and capsaicin cream would be valuable.

Tricyclic antidepressants (at a median dose of 50 mg at night) have been shown to be effective in post-surgical breast pain. Capsaicin 0.075% is successful in the treatment of post-mastectomy pain. Topiramate has been described as of use in isolated intercostal neuralgia.

Further reading

Macrae WA. Chronic pain after surgery. British Journal of Anaesthesia 2001; 87: 88–98.

Related topics of interest

Anatomy and physiology (p. 5); Complex regional pain syndromes (p. 60); Sympathetic nervous system and pain (p. 202).

NEUROMODULATION – TENS, ACUPUNCTURE AND LASER PHOTOBIOMODULATION

These therapies all influence the spinal gate mechanism, reducing pain transmission by neuromodulation and/or biomodulation with gene expression. All have high safety profiles, in trained hands.

Transcutaneous electrical nerve stimulation (TENS)

Transcutaneous electrical stimulation of peripheral nerves through intact skin is effective in controlling some pains. The current is generated by a portable battery-operated device attached to electrodes on the skin. Generally the four-pad units are the most flexible to use. Typically pulses of 50–150 Hz and currents of 15–35 mA are effective. These settings stimulate low-threshold afferents (Aβ mechanoreceptors) causing inhibition of the passage of high-threshold pain fibre impulses (Aδ and C fibres) at the spinal cord level. This is thought to be via presynaptic γ-amino butyric acid (GABA) inhibition of the substantia gelatinosa cell excitation in the spinal gate. High-frequency current selectively stimulates larger afferent fibres. It may also increase the refractory period and reduce firing rate in smaller afferent pain fibres. High-frequency TENS has mainly a segmental effect. Low-frequency stimulation (Aδ mechanism) can produce analgesia in patients who have failed to respond to the more conventional high-frequency stimulation. This is thought to work by activating inhibitory descending neuronal influence in the dorsal horn of the spinal cord.

TENS is applied around the painful area, or along dermatomes relevant to the area, or on related segments paraspinally. Patients should be encouraged to experiment with a variety of settings on the TENS machine (frequency, pulse width, pattern of stimulation) to achieve benefit.

Uses

A systematic review has shown TENS to reduce pain and improve the range of movement in chronic low-back pain patients. TENS is significantly better than placebo in reducing pain and stiffness in osteoarthritis of the knee. Hand pain and joint tenderness is decreased in rheumatoid arthritis.

A trial of TENS is appropriate for most pains which have some nociceptive element. TENS has been effective in treating facial pain, myofascial pain, mechanical back pain, post-amputation pain, refractory angina, mild post-herpetic neuralgia and peripheral nerve injury (particularly where there is paraesthesia).

TENS can be helpful in visceral, neuropathic or metastatic pain of cancer. Twenty-five per cent of radicular pain responds to TENS.

Practicalities

TENS electrode pads need even contact with the skin to minimize current density. This is achieved by good adhesion of the pads and a conducting gel layer underneath the pads. Pads can be self-adhesive or fixed with separate adhesive tape. TENS should be used for at least 30 min, but it can be used for up to 8 h a day if helpful. Most patients gain relief *only* while the machine is switched on. A minority experience relief beyond the period of use. Sites of application should be rotated to avoid skin irritation. Occasionally adhesive allergy occurs and this can be solved by changing the make of pads. For radicular pain, electrode pads are placed over the dermatomal distribution of the affected nerve.

Constant high-frequency stimulation is the normal mode of use, commonly 70–100 Hz. Some patients respond to stimulation at a frequency of 2–4 Hz (acupuncture-like TENS); this requires higher intensity and may cause uncomfortable muscle contractions. Some machines therefore have a modulation facility that allows switching of current and frequency at short intervals.

Limitations

TENS has few side effects.

It is wise to avoid its use in patients with cardiac pacemakers. In pregnancy its use is generally avoided until the onset of labour, especially along dermatomes that innervate the pelvis. TENS works when the normal integrity of the sensory system is maintained, and is thus of little value in the presence of cutaneous numbness or states of hypersensitivity in which the Aβ fibres are stimulating rather than inhibiting the gate mechanisms of the spinal cord. In addition there is the possibility that skin damage from overstimulation might be missed if the skin is insensitive. Electrodes should not be applied to an insensate area, as titration of stimulus is not possible and high settings may potentially lead to scorching. They should also not be applied to the anterior triangle of the neck, lest they affect the carotid sinus or recurrent laryngeal nerve. Placement across the cranium is contraindicated. This avoids the possible risk of an induced epileptic event. TENS is impractical while asleep and potentially dangerous when driving (in case of sudden increased stimulus intensity secondary to electrode movement). Patients may encounter difficulty in placing electrodes at awkward sites.

Acupuncture

Acupuncture is an ancient Chinese art which has been increasingly practised in the West over the last 25 years. Traditionally its mechanism of action is explained by restoring a balance of energy factors (yin and yang) along intangible body meridians.

Historically and culturally it made a coherent theory. Readers will not be surprised at the absence of a scientific evidence base to support this theory. On the other hand there is an anatomical basis for traditional acupuncture: acupuncture points are close to neuromuscular junctions on muscles or points where nerves penetrate fascial layers. There is also a physiological basis: its effects are explained mainly by segmentally/polysegmentally induced neuromodulation at the spinal and supraspinal level. Acupuncture needles locally traumatize the tissues through which they pass, setting up a small volume of inflammatory mediators (prostaglandins, histamine, bradykinin, leukotrienes, lymphokines, etc.). These stimulate the local nerve endings, the latter for some days. High-threshold mechanoreceptors are activated by the low-frequency high-intensity stimulation. Generated Aδ nerve traffic to the spinal gate is thought to produce enkephalinergic postsynaptic inhibition of the substantia gelatinosa cells. Further spread of this traffic through the crossed spinothalamic tract up to the periaqueductal grey leads to increased descending inhibition of the spinal gate, via fibres from the nuclei raphe magnus and gigantocellularis. Systemic changes of enkephalins and endorphins after acupuncture have been demonstrated. All the effects of acupuncture are reversed by naloxone. Like TENS, acupuncture relies on the integrity of the sensory system: it has no effect if needles are placed in insensate areas.

Electroacupuncture (EA) is the augmentation of the mechanical needle stimulus by using electricity. It can also be used to deliver TENS-like EA at higher frequencies.

Uses

Acupuncture is practised by medical, physiotherapist, complementary and traditional practitioners. Acupuncture is difficult to assess with randomized controlled trials (RCTs), because of the difficulty in selecting a true placebo treatment, as patients are aware of when needles are used.

Attempts to circumvent this problem using 'sham' acupuncture points are likely to be complicated by the observation that any noxious stimulation may activate supraspinal 'diffuse noxious inhibitory controls'. This phenomenon may confound any specific effect of acupuncture and make it particularly difficult to assess the result of a well-designed trial. Claims have been made that the true treatment effect of acupuncture is underestimated as a consequence. Given this limitation it has to be conceded that good-quality studies are in short supply. Recent systematic reviews show evidence of short-term useful pain relief in low-back pain and support its use in idiopathic headaches, but there is also evidence from less rigorously controlled studies. Better evidence is available for its use for antiemesis. It remains a popular treatment in pain clinics. The opportunity to use the window afforded by a short-term response to acupuncture to reduce and discontinue unhelpful or expensive drug treatment is in the opinion of some practitioners a cogent reason for practising acupuncture. The high therapeutic index, assuming of course an understanding of anatomy, is said to justify its widespread use.

This is an oversimplification that fails to take into consideration the negative effects on self-efficacy that may occur with regular and repeated visits to a health professional for a treatment with a short duration of effect. Similarly, the economic benefit of reduction of medication has to be balanced against the cost of providing a professional to undertake the treatment. Exactly the same issues can arise from repeat facet or epidural injections with only short duration of effect, but with the added costs of theatre time.

Practicalities

Asepsis is important. Single-use disposable needles avoid the cross-infection risks of the past. Infected skins areas should be avoided. Around 10% of patients are sensitive to the systemic effects of acupuncture, overtreatment initially causing drowsiness some 6 hours after treatment. Ten per cent of needles induce minor skin bruising.

Major serious side effects are extremely rare. These include pneumothorax, cardiac tamponade, visceral damage, neural damage, blood vessel damage and compartment syndromes in the lower limb. *All* are easily avoidable with knowledge of anatomy. This also allows analysis of the dermatomes, myotomes and sclerotomes affected by needle insertions through skin, muscles or onto periosteum. This forms the basis of Western segmental acupuncture.

Limitations

Repeat treatments are needed to induce pain relief and maintain it. An absolute contraindication is patient refusal. It is relatively contraindicated in patients on anticoagulants. If within anticoagulant range, then superficial needling of skin and superficial muscle has proved to be safe under medical supervision.

There is a place for acupuncture in pain clinics. Its precise role remains difficult to establish. Short-term gains are the rule, and demand for an exotic and unusual treatment must not replace good clinical judgement and its appropriate use alongside other therapies designed to maximize rehabilitation potential and self-efficacy.

Low-level laser therapy (LLLT) – photobiomodulation

Laser therapy in pain work does not involve the high-powered heat-generating (class 4) lasers used in surgery.

The non-thermal application of red and infrared (IR) laser light (class 3B lasers) to tissue has a selective stimulatory effect on *impaired* cells within it. Light in this range penetrates tissue several centimetres. Typical wavelengths used are 810–840 nm (near-IR laser) or 640–670 nm (red light-emitting diodes (LEDs)). Power outputs are 200–1000 mW for near-IR lasers and 10–30 mW for red LEDs. Treatment lengths vary from 30 seconds to 6 minutes, depending on the power used. The laser's effects are better if the light is pulsed onto the tissues (typical range 20 Hz to 5 kHz).

The mechanism of action is at a cellular level. The photons are absorbed directly by mitochondria. The terminal enzyme in the electron transport chain is cytochrome c oxidase. It has four photoacceptor centres that absorb the red and near-IR light, increasing ADP to ATP conversion. This is turn leads to improved cell membrane pump and receptor function, increased cell metabolism, gene expression, and DNA and RNA synthesis. Optimally functioning cells with high intracellular energy stores are unaffected.

Modulation of various biological functions in cell culture and animal models has been shown. In wound healing, cellular proliferation, release of growth factors, increased collagen synthesis and angiogenesis occur. Diffusible growth regulators have been shown to block sensory nerve growth into wounds. Macrophage and lymphocyte stimulation has been demonstrated. Up-regulated cytochrome oxidase activity occurs in cultured neuronal cells.

The laser's action in pain modulation is postulated to be multifactorial:

- A reduction in inflammatory and pain-producing substances in the tissue.
- A normalization of nerve inputs and their membrane function, thereby reducing pain transmission at the spinal gate.
- A secondary phase consisting of the release of endorphins and adrenocorticotrophic hormone (ACTH), which have been shown to be released in man.

Uses

Photobiomodulation (LLLT) has been successfully used in a wide variety of painful conditions, in varying doses (power, time, wavelength, pulsed frequency). It is easier to produce a true placebo laser as a control. Consequently there is better-quality evidence for its use, though variation on energy dosage in clinical trials makes interpretation more difficult.

Systematic review of LLLT in chronic joint disorders shows reduced pain and improved health status; however, varying methodology of application has suggested caution in its interpretation. In rheumatoid arthritis, a systematic review suggests it should be considered for short-term relief of pain and morning stiffness. A systemic review of LLLT in subacute and chronic tendinopathy showed a pooled mean effect of 21–32% pain reduction over placebo. It has been shown to reduce both the intensity and distribution of pain in post-herpetic neuralgia of at least 6 months' duration, which was unresponsive to other methods of treatment.

LLLT has been used in the treatment of many painful conditions: post-traumatic pain of the spine or limbs, failed back surgery syndrome, musculoskeletal pain and chronic post-surgical pains. Less rigorously controlled studies suggest benefit from treating relevant sympathetic ganglia. The author has successfully treated diabetic peripheral neuropathy, resistant to conventional therapies.

Limitations

LLLT is not associated with serious adverse reactions. It has a high benefit to risk ratio. If patients are overtreated, minor side effects can include transiently increased pain, nausea, tiredness or euphoria.

Direct irradiation of the eyes must be avoided.

Its use in carcinoma, over the thyroid gland and in patients on immunosuppression is unwise. Caution should be used in patients with photosensitivity reactions.

Further reading

Alexander JR, MacDonald T, Coates W. The discovery of transcutaneous spinal electro-analgesia and its relief of chronic pain. Physiotherapy 1995; 81(11): 653–61.

De Broucker T, Cesaro P, Willer JC, Le Bars D. Diffuse noxious inhibitory controls in man. Involvement of the spinoreticular tract. Brain 1990 113(4): 1223–34.

Eells JT, Wong-Riley MTT, VerHoeve J et al. Mitochondrial signal transduction in accelerated wound and retinal healing by near-infrared light therapy. Mitochondrion 2004; 4: 559–67.

Ernst E, White A. Acupuncture: safety first. British Medical Journal 1997; 314: 1362.

Hashimoto T, Kemmotsu O, Otsuka H, Numazawa R, Ohta Y. Efficacy of laser irradiation on the area near the stellate ganglion is dose dependent: double-blind crossover placebo-controlled study. Laser Therapy 1997; 9: 7–12.

Moore KC, Hira N, Kumar PS. Double blind crossover trial of low level laser therapy in the treatment of post herpetic neuralgia. Laser Therapy 1988; 1: 7–9.

Systematic reviews

Bjordal JM, Couppé C, Chow RT, Tunér J, Ljunggren EA. A systematic review of low level laser therapy with location-specific doses for pain from chronic joint disorders. Australian Journal of Physiotherapy 2003; 49: 107–16.

Bjordal JM, Couppé C, Ljunggren EA. Low level laser therapy for tendinopathy. Evidence of a dose-response pattern. Physical Therapy Reviews 2001; 6: 91–9.

Brosseau L, Welch V, Wells G, et al. Low level laser therapy (Classes I, II and III) for treating rheumatoid arthritis (Cochrane review). In: The Cochrane Database of Systematic Reviews 1998, Issue 4.

Brosseau L, Welch V, Wells G, et al. Low level laser therapy (Classes I, II and III) for treating osteoarthritis (Cochrane review). In: The Cochrane Database of Systematic Reviews 2004, Issue 3.

Brosseau L, Yonge KA, Robinson V, et al. Transcutaneous electrical nerve stimulation (TENS) for the treatment of rheumatoid arthritis in the hand (Cochrane review). In: The Cochrane Database of Systematic Reviews 2005, Issue 3.

Enwemeka CS, Parker JC, Dowdy DS, et al. The efficacy of low-power lasers in tissue repair and pain control: a meta-analysis study. Photomedicine and Laser Surgery 2004; 22(4): 323–9.

Furlan AD, van Tulder MW, Cherkin DC, et al. Acupuncture and dry needling for low back pain (Cochrane review). In: The Cochrane Database of Systematic Reviews 2005, Issue 1.

Khadilkar A, Milne S, Brosseau L, et al. Transcutaneous electrical nerve stimulation (TENS) for chronic low-back pain (Cochrane review). In: The Cochrane Database of Systematic Reviews 2005, Issue 3.

Lee A, Done ML. The use of nonpharmacological techniques to prevent nausea and vomiting: a meta-analysis. Anesthesia and Analgesia 1999; 88(6): 1362–9.

Melchart D, Linde K, Berman B, et al. Acupuncture for idiopathic headache (Cochrane review). In: The Cochrane Database of Systematic Reviews 2001, Issue 1.

Osiri M, Welch V, Brosseau L, et al. Transcutaneous electric nerve stimulation for knee osteoarthritis (Cochrane review). In: The Cochrane Database of Systematic Reviews 2000, Issue 4.

Related topic of interest

Anatomy and physiology (p. 5).

NEUROMODULATION – SPINAL CORD, PERIPHERAL NERVE AND BRAIN STIMULATION

The recent use of electrical stimulation to relieve pain dates back to 1967, when spinal cord stimulation (SCS) was first attempted by Shealy and co-workers, the logic for this following on from Melzack and Wall's gate control theory for pain published in 1965.

Methods and sites

The commonest site for stimulation for pain is the spinal cord. Stimulation can also be delivered to sites within the brain (such as the thalamus) or occasionally over the motor cortex of the brain. Stimulation can be used for control of conditions other than pain, such as spasticity, bladder control in multiple sclerosis (MS), peripheral vascular disease (PVD) and angina. There is increasing interest in peripheral nerve stimulation for pain – sacral nerve stimulation for incontinence is well evidenced and more recently occipital nerve stimulation is gaining acceptance for occipital neuralgia, cluster headache and even migraine. This growth reflects in part improvements in technology – hitherto, systems able to deliver peripheral nerve stimulation have been unreliable.

TNS (transcutaneous stimulation) is considered elsewhere (previous chapter) in this book. As a form of spinal cord stimulation, it is less invasive than the techniques considered here.

Spinal cord

Physiology

The mechanism of spinal cord stimulation is unknown. Three possible mechanisms have been suggested. Stimulation using currents, voltages and frequencies typically in use is shown to activate the dorsal column fibres. Larger fibres are preferentially activated, though the spinal sympathetic pathways are also activated.

- In the first of these mechanisms it is suggested that antidromic activation of dorsal column fibres 'closes the gate'. This was the original logic behind the development of the use of SCS. This mechanism – modified by current thinking regarding the operation of the gate – may be the most important. In chronic pain states this system is sensitized – hence the phenomena of allodynia and hyperalgesia and the concept of 'wind-up' referred to elsewhere in this volume. There is a failure of γ-amino butyric acid (GABA)-mediated inhibition, and it seems that this is reversed by spinal cord stimulation.

- The second mechanism involves supraspinal pathways. Stimulation passes up the dorsal columns to the anterior pretectal nuclei in the brain stem, and is relayed back down to the spinal cord via the dorsal longitudinal funiculus, where the pain pathways are modulated.
- Lastly, spinal cord stimulation acts by stimulating adrenergic sympathetic neurones. This probably accounts for the effects on blood flow seen in PVD and angina, and on bladder function seen in MS.

However none of these mechanisms has been proven, and all may be important. The effects on blood flow seem separate from the effects on pain. The dorsal columns are important, as pain relief is not obtained unless paraesthesiae are produced in the affected area; indeed the precise position of the electrode is crucial to success of the technique. The observation that paraesthesiae must be perceived by the patient argues for a supraspinal mechanism. Some studies have been made of neurochemical changes resulting from SCS; most of these are inconsistent, though rises in noradrenaline, substance P and 5HT (5-hydroxytryptamine) have been observed. In contrast to TNS, the action of SCS is unaffected by naloxone.

Methods

An electrode array is positioned over the midline of the spinal cord in the epidural space. The usual minimum surface area of the electrodes is about 6–8 mm^2. At least two electrodes of opposite polarity are required, but it is more usual to use an array of four or more electrodes. The current trend is to use an increasing number of electrodes. There must be at least one electrode of each polarity but thereafter any combination of polarity and number of electrodes in use is possible. The electrodes are activated in one of two ways. The more usual practice is to connect the electrodes to a battery-powered internal transmitter. The alternative is to use a receiver implanted subcutaneously (usually the flank). This receiver is powered by induction from an external transmitter, using an aerial attached to a battery-powered transmitter. However these systems are becoming less and less used. The fully internal systems do not require the patient to continuously have a receiver taped to the body; this allows much more freedom of activity – especially when sleeping, or in daily activities. The disadvantage is that the battery must be renewed periodically – usually about every 3–5 years depending on use.

The system can be programmed in detail; programmable parameters include varying frequency of stimulus, amplitude, duration of stimulus pulse and which electrode in the array is active and its polarity.

During the preparation of this volume a new generation of technologies was being introduced, which represents the first technological advance in the field for many years. The new equipment has more complex electrode arrays, more complex programming functionality and percutaneously rechargeable batteries – these being necessary to cope with the increased current demands of the newer systems. The logic is that with an increased number of electrodes and programming possibilities – independent and multiple polarities – increased efficacy will be obtained, thus extending the indications (in particular for the back pain component of failed back surgery).

Surgical procedure

Electrodes can be implanted percutaneously, or at open operation. Whatever the method, positioning of the electrode is crucial – although the newer technology electrodes and programming capabilities aim to overcome this by providing more flexibility. Paraesthesiae must be elicited in the area of the pain, and there should not be overstimulation of areas unaffected by pain, as such stimulation can prove unpleasant – again a target of the newer technologies. As frequency, pulse width and amplitude of stimulus increase, so does the area covered.

Percutaneous method

Percutaneously the electrode is passed down a Tuohy needle into the epidural space. Current designs mean this electrode must be cylindrical so that the electrode contacts run in a line. Once the electrode is in position, the remainder of the system can be implanted making a subcutaneous tunnel from the back round to the flank where the receiver is usually positioned. The whole procedure can be carried out under local anaesthetic. The advantage of this system is that it is less invasive, and, because it is carried out under local anaesthetic, the correct position of the electrode can be confirmed by stimulation during the procedure. The major disadvantage is that it is difficult to keep such electrodes in a constant position, and this is particularly true in the neck. Movement may then result in sudden and unpredictable decreases or increases in stimulation; the latter are extremely unpleasant for the patient. The method is used when the patient is unfit for general anaesthesia (e.g. SCS for angina), or when expertise necessary to carry out surgical implantation is unavailable.

Surgical implantation

An open operation under general anaesthesia, and partial laminectomy is required when surgical electrodes are to be implanted. Position is held much better, and because a larger electrode surface is available the system provides better and more controllable stimulation. Accurate positioning of the electrode relies upon information from a preoperative trial, or from placing an electrode with a large enough array so that a given combination of electrodes will stimulate the desired area. If electrodes are placed in a partly transverse direction, then two or more electrodes can be programmed from the four available in most arrays to stimulate the desired area.

Trial procedures

Because a major procedure may be involved, and because the stimulator equipment is quite costly, many practitioners will undertake a trial of stimulation prior to permanent implantation. An electrode is passed into the epidural space under local anaesthesia using a Tuohy needle and brought out through the skin to an external power source. The position of the electrode can be adjusted at stimulation and also by staged withdrawal in the ward. The trial normally lasts 5–7 days, but can under certain circumstances last several weeks. It may be necessary to send the patient home to ensure an accurate trial; this may be particularly important in Raynaud's disease as the subject may need to experience a cold environment to provoke the symptoms!

The trial procedure is most useful where predictors of success are low. Many omit the trial stage.

In treating any form of chronic persistent pain it is important that a diagnosis is made. It is important that treatable conditions are not missed (e.g. unrecognized recurrent prolapse of disc following back surgery), and in addition one of the best predictive indicators for successful stimulation is the diagnostic category.

Some of these categories prove difficult to treat for technical reasons. For example it is difficult to achieve effective stimulation of midline areas such as the perianal area; however, when stimulation is obtained, pain relief can be excellent. Another problem in such cases is unwanted excessive stimulation in surrounding areas. Another area which is difficult to access is the head and neck, particularly the scalp.

Attention is also drawn to the failed back surgery syndrome. There continues to be enthusiasm for the treatment of the back pain elements of the condition by SCS although the success rate is poor (Table 1); no trials exist to confirm efficacy. However SCS does prove effective for the leg pain elements of the condition. Improvements in technology may tip the balance in favour of spinal cord stimulation – furthermore it is unclear whether intrathecal opioid therapy may be more or less appropriate in this situation.

Since it is a non-destructive technique, SCS should be used in preference to destructive techniques (e.g. dorsal root entry zone (DREZ) lesions) even if the chance of success is less, since most destructive techniques have a high delayed relapse rate, and may cause neurological deficit. Consequently, it is reasonable practice to perform a trial of SCS for brachial plexus avulsion pain prior to DREZ although it nis unlikely to be successful. As a low-risk procedure, trial of SCS is worth considering prior to intracranial procedures for central post-stroke pain.

Case selection

Case selection may be considered under four headings: diagnosis, influences on the pain, response to trial and psychological assessments and adjuvant therapy.

Diagnosis (as discussed above).

Influences on the pain. Most of these can be elucidated in the history in outpatients. If the pain is susceptible to external influence it is more likely to respond to spinal cord stimulation. Examples are the response of the pain to changes in temperature, to rubbing, to transcutaneous stimulation and to distraction. A reduction in pain indicates a high chance of stimulation being effective. Increase in pain due to allodynia can also predict a good response, though this is not as hopeful a predictor as when there is pain relief. Some early

Table 1. Success rates for SCS

Indication	Success rate
Angina	Almost certain response
Ischaemic limb pain	
Causalgia, regional pain syndrome	Success rate ~70–80%
Reflex sympathetic dystrophy	
Peripheral nerve lesion*	
Brachial plexus damage*	
Cauda equina damage*	
Nerve root avulsion*	
Amputation stump pain	
Painful diabetic peripheral neuropathy	
Leg pain after failed back surgery syndrome	
Back pain after failed back surgery syndrome	Moderate success ~40–50%
Arachnoiditis	
Partial spinal cord lesion	
Phantom limb pain	
Post-herpetic neuralgia	
Nociceptive pain, including cancer	Low chance of success
Central post-stroke pain	
Vaginal, penile and perianal pain	
Intercostal neuralgia	
Facial anaesthesia dolorosa	Do not respond
Atypical facial pain	
Complete cord lesion	
Abdominal pain	

*If there is nerve injury with preserved, though disordered sensation (dysaesthesia), then success is likely; if there is established neurological deficit, then response is unlikely.

work suggests that if during a trial there is a reduction in the area of allodynia success is likely. Using these clinical criteria, those with positive features produce an excellent outcome after permanent stimulation in approximately 60% of cases.

Response to trial. A positive response indicates a high likelihood of success, though not a certainty. In the audit referred to below a positive trial predicted a 90% chance of success (86% excellent outcomes); however it is not perfect and 10% of responders ultimately prove failures.

Psychological assessments and adjuvant therapy. Increasingly the view is taken that a formal assessment should be undertaken prior to implantation and that pain management techniques can be employed with benefit alongside stimulation.

It can be seen that the percutaneous trial is particularly important in the groups where success is predicted to be 40–50% or less. SCS is one of a number of treatments that could be used for certain conditions, although it will be clear from the above that there are some conditions in which its use is indicated if less-invasive treatments fail. Where the chance of success is small, there are as yet no clear criteria to direct the choice of therapy between, say, SCS and other expensive and invasive procedures such as implantable intrathecal drug delivery systems. Extreme caution in assessing developments in this area is advised.

Outcome

There is now a strong evidence base for both the efficacy and effectiveness of this therapy. A number of randomized controlled trials have now been published and in addition an economic analysis found SCS to be cost-effective. Spinal cord stimulation was shown to be more effective than reoperation for failed back surgery; and SCS with physical therapy more effective than physical therapy alone in complex regional pain syndromes (CRPS). A number of case series have looked at long-term outcome and show there is a reduction in success rate with time, although a reasonable expectation is that 60–70% of patients will experience more than a 50% reduction of their pain 5 years after implantation. In one study return to work was demonstrated and in another increased mobility was shown using external motion sensors attached to joints.

Postoperative management and follow up

Following successful implantation good results are obtained only when there is adequate follow up. This is optimally achieved by a specialist nurse and dedicated physiotherapist running 'neuromodulation clinics' with the implanting neurosurgeon. There should be support available from other pain specialists. Multidisciplinary input is necessary for all but the most straightforward of cases. It may help to know that in many series the revision rate is quite high, anywhere between 25 and 50% of implants requiring surgical revision, and the use of battery-powered implantable devices means replacement will be required every 3–5 years. The fact that this is necessary is some demonstration of the long-term efficacy of the treatment.

SCS indications for vascular disease: the pain of vascular disease

SCS is extremely effective in treating these conditions. The action seems to be different from that of pure pain relief in that the mechanism appears to be an inhibition of the descending sympathetic pathway in the spinal cord. This is believed to prevent sympathetically mediated vasoconstriction. Supraspinal pathways are probably not involved and are certainly less important than in simple pain relief.

Angina

SCS is effective in over 80% of cases. There is excellent pain relief, and the patient's usage of GTN (glyceryl trinitrate) declines. The inhibition of sympathetic vasoconstriction also appears to improve myocardial function, and there is increasing evidence that this is the route by which pain relief is produced. At higher exercise levels the patients still experience angina, so this is not felt to be an unsafe treatment. In uncontrolled studies, survival seems to be improved compared with predictions from actuarial tables.

PVD

SCS is highly effective in treating the pain of intermittent claudication due to peripheral vascular disease. It is more effective in the early stages of the disease. Increases in skin temperature, signals from laser Doppler and transcutaneous oxygen measurements occur with stimulation. This is a consequence of sympathetic system inhibition. There is, however, no evidence for an increase in muscle blood flow. Overall, 80% of patients notice an improvement in pain control; 65% an improvement in walking distance and in 30% this improvement will be significant. These percentages improve if end-stage disease is excluded. Improvements in ulcer healing are also claimed and there may be a reduction in the amputation rate. Unlike the case of angina, it appears that the effect on pain is separate from that on flow, as stimulating at higher levels in the spine (T8 vs T12) is still effective. SCS can help in vasospastic conditions such as Raynaud's disease. It is worth trying in diabetics although the response rate is not as good due to the multiplicity of problems, both vascular and neuropathic.

Diabetic neuropathy

Painful diabetic neuropathy can be difficult to treat. However in a small series of 10 cases assessed by trial stimulation, 8 patients responded at the trial stage and were implanted. Of these, 6 patients obtained long-term relief (follow up 3 years); 1 patient did not and 1 patient died from an unrelated cause. There was relief of both the neuropathic pain and increase in exercise tolerance.

Multiple sclerosis

Approximately 25% of cases of multiple sclerosis experience some form of central pain syndrome. These syndromes may respond to SCS. An additional benefit is that improvements in bladder control may result in up to 70–80% of patients.

Deep brain stimulation

Indications

Severe chronic pain in the face, arms or legs is often due to partial nerve injury such as may occur in amputation or stroke. Deep brain stimulation can be used in cases of central post-stroke pain. Many patients will be reluctant to undergo this form of surgery for a chronic pain condition; it is of course the case that any procedure invasive to the brain carries risk of stroke and to life, albeit very small. Invariably the patient will have found other methods, including trial of SCS, to be ineffective.

Methods

Under local anaesthetic a burr hole is made in the skull and an electrode passed stereotactically to the intended target, normally within the thalamus, though some have tried other sites such as periaqueductal grey matter. A trial of stimulation is performed to make sure the electrode is in the desired physiological target, and then a trial of the therapeutic effect over a few days. After a few days, and provided the trial is successful, a permanent device is implanted and connected to this electrode. The technique originally fell out of favour because of problems with electrode design but has been revisited recently with improvements in electrode design (mainly motivated by an increase in deep brain stimulation for movement disorders). A trial stage is required because a significant number of patients will turn out to be non-responders and a stimulator inappropriate.

Outcomes

Perhaps only 50% of patients will respond and be implanted. The overall conclusion is that this technique is unproven.

Motor cortex stimulation

Indications

The main indication is for central post-stroke pain where the referred area in which the pain is felt is the upper limb or face. The leg motor cortex is difficult to target being mainly in the interhemispheric fissure; it is also difficult to target a large area hence it cannot be considered when the syndrome covers half the sensorium.

Methods

A craniotomy is performed and electrodes placed over the motor cortex. Intraoperative neurophysiology and/or sophisticated image guidance techniques may be necessary to locate the part of the brain which is the motor cortex. The common practice now is to obtain a functional magnetic resonance imaging (fMRI) scan in which the motor cortex has been localized; to employ intraoperative frameless stereotactic neuronavigation techniques to facilitate placement of an electrode. The final placement is confirmed by neurophysiological methods – direct motor cortex stimulation and recording of the somatosensory evoked response. A trial is performed before a permanent device is used, as the percentage of patients who turn out to be responsive to this form of therapy is small. If the cortex is stimulated too vigorously there is a risk of seizures. Unlike stimulation of the sensory pathways there are no paraesthesiae to indicate function of the stimulator, so overstimulation is a real risk. Since it is an intracranial procedure there must also be risk of stroke (and therefore to life) from haemorrhage or infection and a risk of epilepsy, however low these risks must be.

Outcomes

These have not been uniformly encouraging, so currently the method should be regarded as unproven. However using the technology mentioned above it has been possible to more accurately and reliably target the motor cortex, which has led in turn to more optimistic reports in the literature. It has been realized with the advent of fMRI that there is sufficient plasticity of the nervous system that the position of the motor cortex may not be as predicted anatomically following stroke. However, there is impetus behind development of such techniques as they represent an option of medical management for a minority of patients who have failed all other treatments.

Further reading

British Pain Society. Spinal cord stimulation for the management of pain: recommendations for best clinical practice 2005.

Buchser E, Paraschiv-Ionescu A, Durrer A, et al. Improved physical activity in patients treated for chronic pain by spinal cord stimulation. Neuromodulation 2005; 8(1): 40–8.

Daousi C, Benbow SJ, MacFarlane IA. Electrical spinal cord stimulation in the long-term treatment of chronic painful diabetic neuropathy. Diabetic Medicine 2005; 22(4): 393–8.

Jacobs MJ, Jorning PJ, Beckers RC, et al. Foot salvage and improvement of microvascular blood flow as a result of epidural spinal cord electrical stimulation. Journal of Vascular Surgery 1990; 12: 354–60.

Kaplitt MG, et al. Deep brain stimulation for chronic pain. In: Winn HR, ed. Youmans Neurological Surgery, 5th edn. Philadelphia: WB Saunders, 2003.

North RB, Kidd DH, Zahurak M, James CS, Long DM. Spinal cord stimulation for chronic, intractable pain: experience over two decades. Neurosurgery 1993; 32(3): 384–95.

Nuti C, Peyron R, Garcia-Larrea L, et al. Motor cortex stimulation for refractory neuropathic pain: four year outcome and predictors of efficacy. Pain 2005; 118(1–2): 43–52.

Rees G. Mechanism of action of spinal cord stimulation. Pain Reviews 1994; 1: 184–98.

Simpson BA. Spinal cord stimulation. Pain Reviews 1994; 1: 199–230.

Taylor RJ, Taylor RS. Spinal cord stimulation for failed back surgery syndrome: a decision analytic model and cost effectiveness analysis. International Journal of Technoogyl Assessment in Health Care 2005; 21(3): 351–8.

Related topics of interest

Back pain – medical management (p. 34); Back pain – surgery (p. 40); Chest pain (p. 56); Complex regional pain syndromes (p. 60); Multiple sclerosis (p. 91); Nerve blocks – infusion techniques in chronic pain (p. 114); Neuromodulation – TENS, acupuncture and laser photobiomedulation (p. 146); Stroke: (p. 199).

NEUROSURGICAL TECHNIQUES

This chapter is not intended as a comprehensive account of all the neurosurgical procedures for pain; rather it is intended to explain the rationale of neurosurgery for pain, and illustrate some of its potential. One of the most important roles of a neurosurgeon involved in surgery for pain is to be certain that surgically remediable pathology has not been missed – in the case of 'chronic' sciatica this may be a simple lumbar disc prolapse – more rarely 'trigeminal neuralgia' may represent the facial pain from an acoustic or even trigeminal schwannoma. As far as specialist pain clinic practice is concerned, procedures may involve quite specialized techniques drawn from different areas of neurosurgery such as spinal neurosurgery or stereotactic and image-guided techniques. The 'pain' neurosurgeon thus requires considerable general and specialist expertise. A fully equipped neurosurgical facility is of course required, with facilities for intraoperative neurophysiological monitoring.

Neurosurgery for the relief of persistent pain began in the 19th century with root sections and later cordotomy. Pain relief was dominated by these methods until the second half of the 20th century when advances in analgesics, including anticonvulsants, psychotropics and specific opiate preparations, were associated with the rapid development of pain clinics and hospices. There was then a virtual cessation in the practice of neurosurgery for pain relief.

In the last 20 years the development of more precise, safe, effective and low-morbidity techniques has resulted in a renewed interest in neurosurgery for the relief of pain when medication has proved inadequate or intolerable. These advances include percutaneous techniques and non-destructive/augmentative techniques such as electrical stimulation or the implantation of sophisticated devices for drug delivery. The percutaneous techniques were particularly suited to an anaesthetic training, from which specialty many pain practitioners came.

The procedures performed are of three types:

> **Correct the pathological cause of the pain.** Microvascular decompression (MVD) for trigeminal neuralgia (TGN), spinal fusions for instability – for example in trauma or in spinal metastatic malignant disease, discectomy, tumour resections – the list is not exhaustive!

> **Non-destructive or augmentative techniques such as electrical stimulation.** These techniques are now commonly grouped together under the heading 'neuromodulation'. At many sites in the nervous system, though most commonly the spinal cord; at its most sophisticated this includes stimulation of deep brain structures. A separate strategy, also regarded as a form of neuromodulation, is the implantation of intrathecal infusion devices. The use of intrathecal baclofen for multiple sclerosis and opioids for cancer depends on a surgically implanted device.

> **Destructive procedures.** Radiofrequency lesioning, root sections, open cordotomy, commissurotomy, dorsal root entry zone (DREZ), medullary tractotomy, thalamotomy and historically pituitary ablation.

In the first category, apart from MVD (see below), the examples may appear at first sight unrelated to the specialty of pain. However most spinal neurosurgeons regard lumbar microdiscectomy as simply a procedure for pain relief.

The distinction between destructive and non-destructive procedures is important since destructive procedures are most appropriate for treatment of persistent pain due to malignancy where life expectancy is limited and are little used for non-malignant pains. The reason for this is that relapse rates are high after destructive procedures; there is a risk of neurological deficit and therefore disability; and new syndromes (particularly dysaesthetic-type pains) may arise after destruction of the nervous system at either peripheral or central levels, though more particularly after peripheral lesions. This is due to plasticity of the central nervous system – the same process by which phenomena such as allodynia arise.

Another underlying and related philosophy is that low-risk procedures are to be attempted before high-risk procedures even if the success rate of the former is poor; thus deep brain lesions or stimulation tend to be last resort options. Finally, it is important that a multidisciplinary approach occurs: this may be achieved by joint ward rounds and clinics between anaesthetic, neurological and neurosurgical pain specialists, and involving nurse specialists, and the pain management team.

Several chapters elsewhere in this book deal in detail with the first and second categories – neurosurgery for spinal problems, neurosurgical procedures for trigeminal neuralgia – are examples of procedures correcting a pathology, and there are also separate accounts of electrical stimulation and intrathecal drug delivery therapy. Accordingly, the remainder of this chapter details the final 'last resort' type surgical treatments – lesions of the central nervous system.

Lesions

It has been mentioned above that lesions for pain are to be avoided because of the risk of pain recurrence: development of late dysaesthetic pains and of course the inevitable loss of function that may occur. An example of this is lesioning the lateral cutaneous nerve of the thigh for meralgia paraesthetica. Although widely practised, the outcomes of this are poor and include all three of the complications mentioned above. One exception is perhaps lesions of the trigeminal ganglion via the foramen ovale (discussed in more detail elsewhere); here, although there is loss of function, there is good pain relief which is maintained in a high percentage of cases, though not all. Two well-known lesioning techniques are now discussed in greater detail. There are a number of destructive lesions of the spinal cord designed to alleviate pain. Of these, procedures such as cordotomy and commissural myelotomy are reserved for cases of cancer. The DREZ lesion is unusual in that it is used for chronic pain due to non-malignant causes. Cordotomy and commissural myelotomy certainly have relapse rates, and like DREZ carry risk of significant physical disability.

Dorsal root entry zone (DREZ) lesion

Historical

It was first introduced by Sindou in 1972 as a treatment for neuropathic pain and spasticity. He coined the term microsurgical selective posterior rhizotomy.

The lesion was also popularized by Nashold in 1976 who used radiofrequency technology to create the lesion in the dorsal root entry zone – hence the acronym 'DREZ', particularly for brachial plexus lesions.

Syndromes

The only indication that has truly stood the test of time is for brachial plexus avulsion injuries; it has also been used for well-localized cancer pain, as in Pancoast's syndrome (carcinoma of the lung apex associated with brachial neuralgia), cauda equina and spinal cord lesions for pain corresponding to segmental lesions, peripheral nerve lesions, amputations and herpes zoster provided the predominant component of the pain is paroxysmal and associated with allodynia. It can also be used for spasticity, and for hyperactive neuropathic bladder. However it is not widely practised for conditions other than brachial plexus avulsions.

Operation

This is an open neurosurgical procedure requiring a laminectomy with opening of the dura to expose the spinal cord. The DREZ region is identified from the position of the dorsal rootlets. A lesion of depth 2–3 mm is created affecting Rexed laminae I–IV. This may be difficult to identify when the roots have been avulsed, as is the case in brachial plexus injuries. There may also be problems in identifying the correct level and intraoperative fluoroscopy can be used. Some clinicians employ intraoperative neurophysiological monitoring of somatosensory evoked potentials in order to guard against unintentional damage to the dorsal columns.

Risks

The main complication is ipsilateral leg weakness, though there may also be ipsilateral loss of sensation. Some subjective loss of sensation and/or weakness may occur in as many as 60% of cases and be significant in up to 10%. Loss of bladder control can occur, albeit rarely. For these reasons DREZ lesion is often only attempted as a last resort; it may follow attempts at spinal cord stimulation, even if this is not thought likely to succeed.

Outcomes

For brachial plexus lesions success rates of 70% are reported with long-term follow up of between 1 and 8 years. Rates of 50–70% are found for other indications; where relief is obtained it does seem to be maintained. However, there is a tendency to relapse with time, a finding in keeping with most other ablative or destructive techniques for the treatment of pain.

Results for post-herpetic neuralgia are much less encouraging; although initial success rates of about 60% are observed, this falls to only 25% with longer follow up.

Cordotomy

Indications

This procedure is performed almost exclusively for malignant pain – classically, for infiltrating pain from Pancoast's syndrome – but also finds use in cases of mesothelioma. The ideal candidate has pain around the torso or into the lower limbs on one side. Bilateral cases can be considered, but significant side effects then accepted.

Methods

Cordotomy can be performed either percutaneously or at open operation. The aim is to cut the anterior spinothalamic tract.

The percutaneous and more commonly performed method is by contralateral cervical puncture between C1 and C2. The procedure is performed under fluoroscopic control. Contrast is injected, which enables the ligamentum denticulatum to be identified so that a radiofrequency needle can be inserted. Stimulation is carried out to confirm hypoalgesia in the desired area (the patient typically experiences a feeling of warmth rather than paraesthesiae) and then a lesion can be made in the spinothalamic tract. This technique is suitable if the level of pain is below C5.

The open method requires a general anaesthetic and a laminectomy above the level of the pain. The spinal cord is exposed, rotated gently using the ligamentum denticulatum and an incision made in the contralateral anterior quadrant to the pain. The depth of the lesion is approximately 2–3 mm, judged by the operator. The procedure is quite simple and of much lower morbidity than the description might suggest, though not competitive to the percutaneous method.

Complications of both methods are ipsilateral muscle weakness. If performed bilaterally, then loss of bladder function should be included. Risk to respiration, particularly if performed at the cervical level, is significant. If performed for chest pain for lung carcinoma, the respiratory function on the side of the pain may already be compromised. Therefore the production of weakness on the 'good' side may be significant. If bilateral cervical lesions are performed, the patient's respiratory centres can be affected, so that 'Ondine's curse' may develop – here respiration only occurs while the patient is awake. This leads to an indication for open, high-thoracic cordotomy when a previous contralateral percutaneous cervical cordotomy has been performed. How high this cordotomy should be must be judged: lower in order to preserve function, but as the fibres may cross over as many as eight levels, too low will result in loss of efficacy.

Results

It is a highly effective, and probably underused method of pain control in patients with advanced carcinoma. It should be accepted that pain relief will last for only a few months. In the context of patients with advanced carcinoma this is acceptable. In addition the patient may already be disabled by the disease so that side effects are also acceptable. Although the procedure has been performed historically for non-cancer pain, this cannot be recommended.

Commissural myelotomy

The spinal cord is divided, thereby cutting the pain fibres as they cross over. The indication is for pelvic pain from advanced carcinoma; it is rarely performed, as a bilateral cordotomy would achieve the same goal in the rare circumstance of failure of medical management. The morbidity is quite high with effectively loss of use of the lower limbs, and bladder and bowel control.

Related topics of interest

Nerve block in cancer pain management (p. 111); Neuralgia – trigeminal and glossopharyngeal (p. 134).

OSTEOARTHRITIS

Osteoarthritis is a common cause of pain and disability, particularly in the elderly. Initially described in respect of its radiological features, oesteoarthritis was seen as a consequence of 'wear and tear' rather than as an active disease process. Recent evidence of ongoing active disease has led to a challenge to this view, and its replacement by a view that osteoarthritis is a complex condition involving the whole synovial joint and adjacent bone.

In osteoarthritis pathological changes are found in articular cartilage, the synovium, joint capsule and the subchondral bone. Peripheral sensitization and central sensitization may be involved in the pathogenesis of pain, which like the accompanying features of stiffness and loss of function, correlate poorly with radiological changes, and indeed may precede them.

The logic of using nonsteroidal anti-inflammatory drugs (NSAIDs) is based on the assumption that the changes of osteoarthritis are associated with active inflammation. This view has been repeatedly challenged, as inflammation is a variable feature and evidence of effectiveness has been limited. The animal model on which the original trials of NSAID mechanisms were performed does not have a human equivalent and is not pathologically similar to osteoarthritis. Despite this, many early trials of NSAIDs were undertaken using osteoarthritis as a human model. Many trials compared different NSAID preparations, but few differences between drugs were found. Some trials compared NSAIDs with placebo, but few compared them with paracetamol, a pure analgesic without anti-inflammatory properties. The evidence in favour of NSAIDs for osteoarthritis pain is tempered by the very real risk of gastrointestinal side effects with prolonged use. The cyclo-oxygenase II inhibitors (COXIBs) have a similar effect as NSAIDs on pain associated with osteoarthritis, but without the gastrointestinal side effects. However, recent evidence on cardiovascular safety has severely limited the usefulness of this class of drugs in the population most at risk of osteoarthritis. Some increased safety may be conferred by the use of topical NSAIDs.

In contrast to the research effort for NSAIDs in osteoarthritis, there has been relatively little coordinated research on the efficacy of other treatments, or indeed on the other features of the pain syndrome associated with osteoarthritis. Fear of movement and fear of severe disease have been separately identified as contributing to the overall disability and preventing the beneficial aspects of exercise and movement. The following is a summary of the available treatments for which reasonable evidence for efficacy has been sought:

- *Acupuncture.* This is commonly used, but studies comparing acupuncture with 'sham' acupuncture, where needles are placed randomly, have been inconclusive.
- *Capsaicin 0.025%.* This is effective for osteoarthritis of the knee.
- *Education* about arthritis and exercises for muscle strengthening around specific joints have been shown to be of value.
- *Glucosamine.* This preparation, whose pharmaceutical status as a food additive or drug has not yet been established, is currently the subject of great interest. Up to 20% of patients derive pain relief and there is some evidence of reduction of joint space narrowing.

- *Joint lavage.* This may be performed with or without injection of steroids or hyaluronic acid: use of both these drugs is supported by randomized controlled trials.
- *Low-level laser therapy (LLLT).* This has been assessed with a systematic review that has identified one controlled trial out of four demonstrating benefit.
- *Transcutaneous electrical nerve stimulation (TENS).* This is effective in osteoarthritis of the knee.

It is thus useful to consider the pain management of osteoarthritis as management of a wider ranging 'pain syndrome'. Clearly there are some patients who present with end-stage joint destruction of weight-bearing joints for which arthroplasty is the logical and obvious treatment of choice, but lesser degrees of radiological change or small-joint arthritis may lend themselves to simpler methods. Overcoming fears about the consequences of movement, for example in respect of joints that display crepitus, is important as a strategy for encouraging the exercise. From the descriptions above, there may be a place for the use of NSAIDs or COXIBs, particularly during periods when pain is more intense, but the side effects have to be considered, and recent guidance on these drugs emphasizes the importance of using them for the shortest possible length of time. The role of treatments such as acupuncture or LLLT that require the input of a professional on a regular and open-ended basis is difficult to establish. There is a risk of 'over medicalization' of a problem, with repeated visits to a health care professional and a risk of spending a large proportion of the week seeking help over a problem that might be better dealt with by encouraging self-sufficiency and exercise and the use of analgesics. The use of paracetamol with or without a weak opioid is logical. Long-acting strong opioids may be indicated, subject to the usual precautions necessary for their use. The purpose of the pharmacological intervention must not be forgotten: the strategy is one of encouraging use of an affected joint by providing adequate analgesia. The use of specific nerve blocks to allow mobilization in the short term may help by providing a patient with the opportunity to demonstrate that a joint is capable of movement.

Further reading

Transcutaneous electrical nerve stimulation for knee arthritis. Cochrane Library, Issue 4, 2000.
Watson MC, Brookes ST, Kirwan JR, Faulkner A. The comparative efficacy of non-aspirin non-steroidal anti-inflammatory drugs for the management of osteoarthritis of the knee: a systematic review. In: Tugwell P, Brooks P, Wells G, et al. (eds). Musculoskeletal Model of the Cochrane Database of Systematic Reviews. The Cochrane Library. The Cochrane Collaboration Issue 1. Oxford: Update Software; 1997.

Related topics of interest

Musculoskeletal pain syndromes (p. 95); Therapy – anti-inflammatory drugs (p. 211); Therapy – capsaicin (p. 219).

PELVIC AND VULVAL PAIN

Gynaecological pain can be considered along with pain affecting the urinary tract because a number of syndromes with non-specific symptoms and overlapping features are described. Common nociceptive mechanisms are implicated. Difficulties in diagnosis of the patient presenting with pain in the lower abdomen may lead to extensive investigation of the genitourinary system. Further confusion may be the consequence of the pain being referred from, or referred to, the musculoskeletal system. Iatrogenic causes may confuse. An empirical approach to symptom control, such as the use of frequent courses of antibiotics for symptoms of pain on micturition, may lead to painful candidiasis.

Investigation may reveal pathology to account for the problem. The indication for, and the possible findings of, investigation is outside the scope of this book. Laparoscopy has improved the diagnosis of painful pelvic pathology but comes with a 1:400 risk of serious complications. As a diagnostic tool it has not answered some essential questions, in the same way that magnetic resonance imaging (MRI) of the spine has not helped the management of many back conditions. The poor correlation between abnormal laparoscopic findings and the symptoms of pain – up to one-third of patients undergoing laparoscopy for pelvic pain have no abnormal findings – together with the inability of the technique to diagnose such conditions as irritable bowel syndrome or stage the degree of endometriosis mean that laparoscopy should not be considered an essential prerequisite to the management of pelvic pain. Indeed there is evidence that patients who are offered laparoscopy as a routine investigation for chronic pelvic pain suffer more pain than those who are offered appropriate treatment based on the clinical interview and examination alone. The implication is that, as with other types of investigation, a negative result may worsen the distress of the patient who is anxious to have a diagnosis. Any attempt to explain how patients with normal pelvic organs continue to experience pain has to consider that an incomplete or erroneous diagnosis may have been made, that the disturbance is physiological rather than pathological, or that psychological factors are playing a part.

Anatomy

The nerve supply to the pelvic viscera is notable for the following:

- The anatomical organization is complicated, with primary afferent nociceptive fibres entering the spinal cord via fibres which pass with efferent nerves of both the sympathetic (thoracic and lumbar spinal nerve roots) and parasympathetic (sacral nerve roots) divisions of the autonomic nervous system.
- The segmental representation of the pelvic afferent is wide. The receptive fields for dorsal horn neurones are large. Pelvic afferents project to the spinal cord between T9 (for ovary) and L1 (for bladder and cervix). Ovarian afferents access the lower thoracic spinal roots via the lumbar sympathetic chain, whereas bladder and cervical afferents access the lumbar roots as the presacral nerves or hypogastric plexi. In both sexes there is identified a number of nerve plexi (named after the target organ) through which the

sympathetic fibres pass to the spinal cord: the distribution of the sympathetic fibres to and from these plexi follows the blood supply to the organ.

The pelvic splanchnic nerves (S2–S4) are parasympathetic sensory and motor to cervix, lower uterine segment, muscular stroma of prostate, distal urethra and bladder. The relative contribution of the two divisions of the autonomic nervous system to nociception in health and disease is unknown.

Some measure of the complexity of the processes involved in the genesis of pelvic pain can be gained from considering the following observations:

- The painful 'phantom pelvis' following pelvic exenteration has been described.
- The environment of the uterine nociceptor is subject to change with the physiological processes of ovulation and menstruation. Afferents are sensitized by prostaglandins and leukotrienes, and become sensitive to pressure or ischaemia when the uterus contracts. Similarly, chemical irritation of the peritoneum sensitizes and stimulates afferents.
- The uterine venous system is unique in its ability to accommodate huge increases in its blood flow in pregnancy. It is a valveless system, in which distension may occur in the upright position. The finding of distended uterine veins at venography (an obsolete technique used prior to the era of laparoscopy) was said to be diagnostic of a specific condition of pelvic congestion, believed to be responsible for pain.

Chronic pelvic pain without obvious pathology (CPPWOP)

This term was historically used to provide a diagnosis of exclusion for those patients who present with certain pain symptoms and findings but in whom laparoscopy failed to provide a pathological diagnosis. The symptoms are a dull symmetrical ache, worse before menses, and the signs of tenderness over the ovarian point, a cyanotic cervix and tender adnexae. Psychological examination has revealed findings of anxiety, feelings of being sexually unattractive, inability to sustain relationships and stressful life events prior to symptoms.

It is helpful to consider the condition as either a psychological disorder in which noxious stimulation plays a part, or a painful physiological disturbance. It is conveniently described as a disorder of the autonomic nervous system in which abnormal afferent activity (nociception) and efferent activity (altered blood flow) coexist.

Management of CPPWOP. Relief from pain is reported with oral contraceptives and nonsteroidal anti-inflammatory drugs (NSAIDs) which prevent the synthesis of prostaglandins, compounds involved in sensitization of the uterine nociceptor. A hypo-oestrogenic state is helpful for the control of the pain of endometriosis and is used for the control of CPPWOP, using progesterone-containing contraceptives such as medroxyprogesterone acetate. Physical interventions in the form of presacral nerve blockade via a percutaneous approach or via an open or laparoscopic surgical approach have been successfully reported. In this technique, sphincter control is preserved as the sacral nerve roots are unaffected. The contribution of psychological factors to the experience of pelvic pain is important to assess. General cognitive/behavioural approaches may be of value, but particular problems with issues involving sexual difficulties may need specialist attention.

A systematic review has analysed the randomized controlled trials for the above treatments and has concluded, from the five well-constructed trials, that medroxyprogesterone acetate is useful during the treatment phase, and that counselling with reassurance from ultrasound scanning improves mood and reduces pain.

Pelvic adhesions

A diagnosis of this pathology can be made at laparoscopy, but a diagnosis cannot explain how some patients with dense adhesions (from pelvic inflammatory disease, endometriosis or previous surgery) have no pain and how some patients are incapacitated with pain despite few findings.

Management. Surgical division of adhesions has a variable success rate. A systematic review concluded that surgery was best reserved for the more serious cases of adhesions.

Dysmenorrhoea

Primary dysmenorrhoea refers to painful periods not associated with pathology. Sensitization of uterine nociceptors is involved in the process. Secondary dysmenorrhoea is described in association with conditions such as endometriosis. The diagnosis of secondary dysmenorrhoea is outside the scope of this book, as is the specific management of the conditions associated with it.

Management. Both oral contraceptives and NSAIDs suppress prostaglandin synthesis and alter the chemical environment of the nociceptor. A hypo-oestrogenic environment is helpful for the prevention of endometriosis: hence the rationale for the use of oral progesterone contraceptives, the androgen danazol and gonadotrophin-releasing hormone (GnRH) analogues in the management of the secondary dysmenorrhoea of endometriosis. Irrespective of any surgery for the pathology itself, pain relief has been achieved by surgical section of the presacral plexus and the uterine nerves.

Systematic reviews have confirmed some benefit from uterine nerve ablation, and a longer-term benefit of presacral neurectomy, but only in respect of primary dysmenorrhoea, not in that of endometriosis. Danazol has been shown to be effective in four trials against placebo for the treatment of the pain of endometriosis. Fifteen trials comparing RnRH analogues with danazol failed to demonstrate a difference between the two classes of drugs in respect of pain relief or modification of disease.

Haematuria/loin pain

The diagnosis is made by exclusion of organic causes to account for recurrent attacks of unilateral or bilateral loin pain associated with haematuria, but not explained by other pathology. Renal biopsy may show a number of features, such as mesangial proliferation, and immune complement C3 deposition in the arterioles, and arteriolar abnormalities may be demonstrated at renal arteriography, but these changes are non-specific and inconsistent. Psychological disturbance may complicate the presentation.

Management. Many approaches have been used for the pain of presumed renal or ureteric origin. Of the more invasive procedures, ureteric catheterization with instillation of a solution of capsaicin into the renal calyx and ureter has been described: this is said to result in a depletion of substance P from the nociceptors of the urothelium. The procedure may require prolonged epidural anaesthesia. Denervation of the kidney by removal of the renal capsule may afford relief, but the long-term results are disappointing. Pain returns or affects the opposite side. Autotransplantation has been reported to achieve good long-term results.

Interstitial cystitis

A history of suprapubic pain, frequency, dysuria and urgency in the absence of infection, and cystometric findings of small bladder capacity and painful catheterization are features of this condition. Cystoscopic findings include petechial haemorrhages and occasionally ulceration. An increase in the number of mast cells in the bladder wall has been noted in sufferers of the condition. The condition occurs predominantly in middle-aged women and may be associated with irritable bowel syndrome. Many patients have had a hysterectomy prior to diagnosis, such that it has been suggested that this operation has been performed because of complaints of pelvic pain that were those of interstitial cystitis.

Management. Steroids and NSAIDs, antihistamines, heparin, long-term antibiotics, local anaesthetics and tricyclic antidepressants have been reported to be of benefit in medical management of interstitial cystitis. Surgical management, with ablation of the vesicoureteric plexus, has been reported to provide long-term relief. Behavioural therapy aimed at reducing the level of distress and associated illness behaviour has been reported to be of value.

Vulvodynia

The International Society for the Study of Vulvovaginal Disease defines vulvodynia as a sensation that is variously described as burning, irritation, rawness or discomfort.

Symptoms may be secondary to pathology such as:

- Dermatitis.
- Human papilloma virus.
- Lichen sclerosis.
- Psoriasis.
- Chronic candida.
- Vulval intraepithelial neoplasia.
- Vulval vestibulitis which affects younger women and causes local dyspareunia. The skin is erythematous and uninfected.
- Dysaesthetic vulvodynia which causes unremitting, burning pain. The histology is normal.

Patients with vulval pain should be seen by a gynaecologist with referral to dermatologists and genitourinary medicine physicians as seen appropriate by the gynaecologist so that causative pathology and otherwise treatable disease has been excluded. Some will have had surgical procedures such as vestibulectomy, skinning vulvectomy or simple vulvectomy which may have exacerbated the pain problem.

Although classification and treatment of vulval pain has not been clearly established, gynaecologists and dermatologists would tend to classify pain as 'with skin changes' or 'without skin changes'. The term dysaesthetic vulvodynia has been suggested to include all pain syndromes of unknown aetiology. There may be some merit in the simple classification of vulval pain into nociceptive and neuropathic categories. Even this apparently simple classification is however confused because words such as dysaesthetic and burning are suggestive of neuropathic pain. However vulval pain can be nociceptive without treatable cause.

For practical purposes pain can be thought of as:

- Nociceptive (due to conditions treated by gynaecologists, dermatologists or genitourinary physicians) or nociceptive with untreatable cause, i.e. vestibulitis (appropriately referred to the pain clinic).
- Neuropathic (appropriately referred to a pain clinic), i.e. 'dysaesthetic vulvodynia' (also termed vulvar dysaesthesia or essential vulvodynia) and pudendal neuralgia.

Nociceptive pain correlates with the category 'vulval pain with visible skin changes' and neuropathic pain with 'vulval pain with absent skin changes'. Neuropathic pain is identified by descriptors such as shooting, burning, stabbing, knife-like and by its signs – painful response to a normally non-painful stimulus such as stroking or garments (allodynia), a heightened response to a painful stimulus (hyperalgesia) and a sensory deficit in the area of pain; the deficit may be subclinical (hyperpathia).

Neuropathic pain can arise from diverse or 'unidentified' nerve damage or specifically from a neuralgia of the pudendal nerve. Allodynia, hyperalgesia and hyperpathia can be demonstrated in areas innervated by the pudendal nerve. Obvious cause, e.g. trauma or infection, may not be identified.

A multidimensional approach to pain management is recommended. Even though the evidence of physical pathology may be impossible to demonstrate, it is important that the patient does not assume a primary psychological explanation to account for it. Vulval pain is thought to bear a relationship to sexual or life stress such as loss of partner, but no relationship to sexual abuse. A full psychosocial assessment, with particular attention to the psychosexual, is warranted.

Acupuncture and transcutaneous nerve stimulation may have a role in the treatment of vestibulitis. NSAIDs/COXIBs and/or simple analgesics may be used. Local anaesthetic creams can be prescribed to cover intercourse.

Neuropathic vulval pain can be treated by antineuropathic medication such as tricyclic antidepressants – nortriptyline 10–25 mg at night or amitriptyline at same dose if agitation or sleep disturbance (average dose for improvement has been reported at 40 mg at night); anticonvulsants – gabapentin 300 mg/day increased weekly by 300 mg up to 1200 mg/day has been shown to be effective. There are reports of successful management of pudendal neuralgia by surgical decompression and by computed tomography (CT)-guided local anaesthetic and steroid injections.

Some workers report that neuropathic pains are sympathetically maintained. These may be amenable to local anaesthetic block of sympathetic chain (ganglion impar block), where pain relief effect will outlast pharmacological duration of local anaesthetic.

Further reading

Jones RW. Vulval pain. Pain Reviews 2000; 7(1).
Kennedy SH, Moore SJ. The initial management of chronic pelvic pain. Guideline 41, Royal College of Obstetricians and Gynaecologists, 2005.

Systematic reviews

Prentice A, Deary AJ, Goldbeck-Wood S, Farquhar C, Smith SK. Gonadotrophin-releasing hormone analogues for pain associated with endometriosis. The Cochrane Library, Issue 4, 2000.
Selak V, Farquhar C, Prentice A, Singla A. Danazol for pelvic pain associated with endometriosis. The Cochrane Library, Issue 4, 2000.
Wilson ML, Farquhar CM, Sinclair OJ, Johnson NP. Surgical interruption of pelvic nerve pathways for primary and secondary dysmenorrhoea. The Cochrane Library, Issue 4, 2000.

Related topics of interest

Musculoskeletal pain syndromes (p. 95); Nerve blocks – sympathetic system (p. 124).

PREGNANCY

Pain in pregnancy is very common and it is important to reassure when appropriate but still recognize potentially serious conditions. The management of pain during labour is beyond the scope of this text.

Pain in pregnancy takes away from what should be an enjoyable experience and pain which goes untreated can result in premature delivery, either spontaneous or induced. The management of pain in pregnancy has to be balanced with fetal well-being. Pains are precipitated either directly or indirectly by pregnancy.

These are due to the mechanical and hormonal effects of pregnancy, due to the modification of other disease by the pregnancy, and due to delivery and procedures undertaken for delivery. Pains of pre-existing conditions may become more symptomatic during pregnancy because treatment has had to be restricted for fetal reasons. A fresh treatment strategy may need to be employed. Because options for treatment are not as plentiful as in the non-pregnant state and because some of these pains are peculiar to the pregnant state, each is given special consideration so therapeutic potential can be maximized. Before deciding on therapies, what is available in terms of fetal safety must be defined.

Treatment

The non-pharmacological methods have an advantage over pharmacological because of fetal safety. If drugs are to be used, non-pharmacological methods may provide dose-reducing adjuncts. Drugs may cover a period in which a non-pharmacological method is getting to work. The first trimester is the time of greatest risk to the developing fetus.

1. Non-pharmacological methods. Physiotherapy can address muscle tension problems, pain problems resulting from altered biomechanics, can facilitate mobilization and can provide sacroiliac belts for the treatment of symphisis pubis diastasis pain, although these are not tremendously helpful.

Transcutaneous electrical nerve stimulation (TENS) is used to treat back pain, pains precipitated by muscle tension, headaches and nerve entrapment. The abdominal wall is avoided as a site for placement of pads to avoid uterine stimulation and the theoretical potential for inducing labour.

Acupuncture is used for the treatment of headache, nerve entrapment pain and back pain. There is a theoretical risk of uterine stimulation but there are no reports of this in the literature.

Water gymnastics (aqua-aerobics) during the second half of pregnancy have been shown to significantly reduce the intensity of back pain.

Stressful social and psychological factors should be addressed.

2. Pharmacological methods. Drugs must be carefully selected and attention given to the timing of the fetus's exposure to the drug. The dose and duration of exposure should be minimized. Because of the ethics of research in pregnancy, there are no controlled studies in pregnant women. The drugs which are used are ones in which animal studies have failed to demonstrate a fetal risk or have shown an adverse effect that was not confirmed in controlled studies in women in the first trimester.

Drugs for which there is positive evidence of human fetal risk and likelihood of causing fetal abnormalities outweighs any benefit should be avoided.

a. Nociceptive pain treatments

- *Paracetamol.* There are no reports of congenital abnormalities attributed to paracetamol. Fetal death has been reported in maternal overdose.
- *Aspirin and nonsteroidal anti-inflammatory drugs (NSAIDs).* The use of these drugs in the third trimester is associated with premature closure of the ductus arteriosus. There is a risk of neonatal haemorrhage, which is of particular concern in the neonate. Low-dose NSAIDs in the second trimester are associated with oligohydramnios. The above risks do not appear to apply to low-dose aspirin as used in pre-eclampsia.
- *Opioids.* Use of codeine in the first trimester has been linked to an increased risk of fetal abnormalities, but recent evidence contradicts this. In the first and second trimesters it is associated with inguinal and umbilical hernias and a neonatal withdrawal syndrome is described.

  Dextropropoxyphene is associated with a neonatal withdrawal syndrome.

  Morphine is safely used for short-term interventions. Most of the available long-term data are for methadone, which is associated with good maternal and fetal outcome and has the advantage of being an NMDA (*N*-methyl-D-aspartic acid) antagonist and therefore having some antineuropathic activity. Long-term users must continue their regular daily dose while in labour. Epidural analgesia may be used for the superimposed pain of labour (including epidural opioids) as tolerance to opioids will be a problem. There will be an increase in analgesic requirements after operative delivery, which can be provided for by epidural or intravenous opioid infusion. Dose equivalents between drugs and routes of administration are unpredictable so the effect of any superimposed analgesic intervention needs to be very carefully monitored.
- *Triamcinolone* (10 mg) in an equal mix of 1% lidocaine and 0.5% bupivacaine up to 20 ml has been used to treat coccydynia, neuromata and nerve entrapment pain.

b. Neuropathic treatments

- *Amitriptyline.* Limb reduction abnormalities have been reported from using amitriptyline in the first trimester. In 500 000 second and third trimester pregnancies there were no reports of fetal abnormalities.
- *Anticonvulsants.* There are no data available for gabapentin but all other anticonvulsants commonly used in pain management are thought to be unsafe.

Breast-feeding

Paracetamol and diclofenac enter breast milk but in such small doses they are thought to be clinically insignificant. Morphine enters breast milk but neonatal effect is limited because of low bioavailability. Amitriptyline enters breast milk and there are reports of neonatal drowsiness which ceases on stopping the amitriptyline.

Management

Multidisciplinary pain management is of importance and medical input should include obstetric and neonatology opinions where necessary. There should be a close link to a psychiatrist as depression is linked to pain and depression is a risk in the postnatal period.

Patients may require management into the postnatal period if their pain persists or even if it has abated for advice as to weaning off their medication and management of potential future problems.

Pains

The management of pain in pregnancy requires the joint input of obstetrician and pain clinician not least so complications of pregnancy can be differentiated from pain syndromes. Reluctance to carry out X-ray investigations should not cause oversight of pain problems of sinister cause such as those due to developing malignancy. Several of the following pains can coexist but each requires separate consideration.

Back pain

An element of back pain is normal during pregnancy. Half of all pregnant patients report back pain at some stage. It results from the lordosis that develops because of the enlarged anterior mass of the uterus. It may also be contributed to by increased laxity in sacroiliac, sacrococcygeal and symphysis pubis joint induced by relaxin. Serious sinister and systemic causes must be excluded. Pre-existing back pain often worsens in severity and frequency of symptoms. Asymptomatic disc herniation is common in pregnancy. 1:10 000 pregnant women will develop radicular symptoms. Spondylolisthesis may be caused by increased joint laxity.

Treatments.   Advice on movement, mobility and lifting should be offered. It has been shown that specially shaped pillows appear to reduce back pain and promote sleep in late pregnancy. Education, support and advice and non-pharmacological methods such as a trochanteric belt and manipulation for sacroiliac pain are used. Paracetamol and opioids can be employed. If radicular pain occurs beyond the first trimester, amitriptyline or epidural triamcinolone may help.

Coccydynia

Coccydynia is associated with alteration in ligament laxity and changes in posture which occur during pregnancy. It is exacerbated by sitting and may be worse in the postpartum period after prolonged sitting during labour. Delivery may cause trauma to the coccyx. There are reports of pre-existing coccydynia being exacerbated by pregnancy. There may be a case in these patients for elective Caesarean section as potential trauma of delivery may exacerbate pain further.

Treatments. Non-pharmacological methods, paracetamol, opioids, injection of steroid to caudal epidural space, coccygeal joints and ganglion impar can be used alone or in combination.

Postpartum back pain

Back pain of pregnancy continues after delivery for longer than 6 months in an estimated 43%. It is worse in the younger multigravid patient with a pre-pregnancy history of back pain.

The relationship of back pain to epidurals is debated. The theory that loss of normal posture and sensation to posture may contribute to the development or exacerbation of back pain has been discounted on the basis that pain is not related to the degree of motor block. The site of epidural puncture can be exquisitely tender in that very localized area. Some have a more widespread area of ache or bruised-like feeling surrounding the point of insertion. The diagnosis of epidural abscess must be excluded.

Treatments for generalized back pain as above; for localized back pain at puncture site, topical NSAIDs, low-level laser therapy.

Physiotherapy should be instituted surrounding the time of epidural blood patching as there are reports of increased backache after the procedure, probably related to immobility.

Symphysis pubis diastasis pain

Relaxation of the pelvic ligaments occurs to allow for more movement of the symphysis pubis. This can occur to the point of widening of the symphysis pubis and instability of the pelvis. There is no evidence however that the degree of symphyseal distraction is related to the amount of pelvic pain. Weight bearing at the symphysis pubis produces movement which is painful, with associated muscle spasm and neuropathic pain caused by tension and pressure on the nerves in the region; sciatica and genitofemoral neuralgia (pain in groin and labia) are associated. The pain often resolves in the few weeks after delivery.

Treatment. TENS, physiotherapy, sacroiliac belts, paracetamol, amitriptyline and opioids are used.

Recurrent loin pain and dysuria without positive microbiology culture

Intermittent loin pain starting in the second or third trimester has been attributed to the enlarging uterus compressing the ureters as they cross the pelvic brim (right side more common than the left). Ureteric dilatation has been demonstrated in the absence of renal stones and the patient gets relief from being on her hands and knees.

Treatment. Heat packs and TENS may be of use. Morphine is used for exacerbations and amitriptyline and diclofenac have been used for prophylaxis.

Diclofenac should be avoided after 34 weeks or if there is any renal compromise.

Upper abdominal pain

Enlargement of the abdomen causes stretching of the abdominal wall which causes both muscular pain and tension on nerves which travel within causing pain. The anterior branches of the anterior rami of the thoracic nerves pierce rectus abdominis. Stretching of rectus abdominis can cause unilateral pain in the distribution of a thoracic nerve extending to the midline. At the point of its emergence from the costal margin the nerve is exquisitely tender. Pain and tenderness are quite common over the edges of the lower ribs where the abdominal muscles insert. Upper abdominal discomfort can also arise from the rounded head of a breech pressing against the ribs. These must be clearly differentiated from upper abdominal pain of pre-eclampsia.

Treatment. Non-pharmacological methods and injection of local anaesthetic and steroid at the point of its emergence from the costal margin may be effective.

Pelvic and lower abdominal pain

Similarly, stretching of the lower abdominal wall can cause pain in the distribution of the iliohypogastric nerve causing pain above the inguinal ligament, ilioinguinal nerve, causing pain in the medial thigh, genitofemoral nerve causing pain in the groin and/or labia, and the lateral cutaneous nerve of thigh causing pain in the lateral thigh (meralgia paraesthetica). Pain is quite often felt in the anterior upper thigh.

Treatment. Non-pharmacological methods and injection to tender points. A neuropathic pain in an area from above pubic bone to above umbilicus has been described. It is thought that this may be a pain maintained by sympathetic supply to the uterus.

Carpal tunnel syndrome

Hand symptoms due to compression of either median or ulnar nerves occur. They are more common in pregnancy because of fluid retention, fat deposition and relaxation of the transverse carpal ligaments by relaxin.

Treatment. Removal of constricting devices, elevation of the limb and the use of splints may help. Surgical release is a last resort.

Headaches

Recurrent headaches tend to improve during pregnancy. They may not however, and patients may be rendered worse because treatment is contraindicated: e.g. sumatriptan is withdrawn because it is known to cause fetal malformations in rabbits. Systemic diseases should be excluded as causes.

Treatment. Non-pharmacological methods should be used if possible. Paracetamol is the mainstay of treatment.

Postdural puncture headache

Treatment. Conservative treatment comprises high oral fluid intake and simple analgesics. Persistent headaches are often treated with an epidural blood patch, with a success rate of 85–90%. This invasive procedure is not free from complications and is contraindicated in patients with meningitis, systemic infection, coagulopathy, cutaneous lumbar lesions and those receiving anticoagulant therapy. Numerous drug therapies have been reported in the literature as alternatives, including sumatriptan, a 5-HT1δ agonist, at a dose of 6 mg subcutaneously and repeated 2 h later and again 9 h later to obtain complete relief.

Neuropraxia

Neuropraxia can be caused by direct needle trauma at the time of regional block or by insertion of the epidural catheter. It can also be caused by birth trauma associated with prolonged labour and cephalopelvic disproportion. It can occur from undue pressure on nerves such as lithotomy position causing trauma to common peroneal nerve, prolonged hip flexion and abdominal oedema causing trauma to the lateral cutaneous nerve of thigh. It is important to exclude an epidural abscess as the cause. Careful examination, early involvement of neurologists and early recourse to MR scanning is important.

Perineal pain and dyspareunia

These conditions can be caused by neuromata or painful swollen scars.

Treatment. Some trials claim a benfit of ultrasound but a systematic review was cautious about the value of this treatment. Other treatments are non-pharmacological, infiltration to scar of local anaesthetic and steroid, amitriptyline and surgical revision if appropriate.

Pain in Caesarean section scar

This pain may be due to trapping of a nerve within layers of scar or due to the development of neuromata. Treatments can be applied as for perineal scars.

Other pains include intractable heart-burn and pain from damage associated with a transient osteoporosis of pregnancy. Back pain and hip pain are common, fractures have been reported during delivery and patients may lose height. It is unclear whether reduction in bone density bears any relationship to pelvic and back pain occurring in pregnancy.

Change in disease due to pregnant state

Rheumatoid arthritis tends to go into remission during pregnancy so the need to prescribe NSAIDs may vanish. Disease-modifying antirheumatic drugs (DMARDs) such as methotrexate and sulfasalazine may be withheld if remission occurs.

Ankylosing spondylitis usually does not change during pregnancy.

Further reading

Roche S, Hughes EW. Pain problems associated with pregnancy and their management. Pain Reviews 1999; 6.

Systematic reviews

Hay-Smith EJC. Therapeutic ultrasound for postpartum perineal pain and dyspareunia (Cochrane review). In: The Cochrane Library, Issue 4, 2000. Oxford: Update software.

Young G, Jewell D. Interventions for preventing and treating backache in pregnancy (Cochrane Review). In: The Cochrane Library, Issue 4, 2000. Oxford: Update software.

PSYCHOSOCIAL ASSESSMENT

Pain is a multifaceted experience and any assessment of it must consider the impact of the pain on the sufferer. Chronic pain is more than a persistent acutely painful condition: it is a condition in which a degree of physiological and psychological maladaptation may occur. Prevention of chronicity is a goal of modern acute pain management, but it is not enough to assume that a simple one-dimensional physical assessment and pharmacological treatment will achieve this. Even in the acute setting it is possible to be aware of presentations that are indicators that a patient is at risk of developing chronic pain. To understand this it is necessary to consider that there are five dimensions to the experience of pain:

- Sensation of pain.
- Suffering and distress: the affective dimension.
- Expectations and beliefs: the cognitive dimension.
- Complaints and non-verbal communication: the behavioural dimension.
- Impact on the patient of the social environment.

Psychosocial 'yellow flags'

Analogous to the 'red flags' in the presentation of back pain which lead the clinician to investigate serious pathology, the 'yellow flags' are symptoms and signs of dysfunction in the psychosocial dimension. A comprehensive assessment that considers carefully the presence of yellow flags is valuable and relevant for the management of acute pain as well as chronic pain. The presence of yellow flags indicates that there may be a problem present at the early stage of an illness that can be managed before the problem, or the way it is addressed by the patient, becomes insoluble. Clearly if yellow flags are to be identified and dealt with at an early stage of the illness, those professionals who take responsibility for early management need to be familiar with the concept and be willing to act upon them: it is not appropriate to expect such factors to wait until secondary care is involved.

A simple scheme for systematic assessment of yellow flags, together with examples of statements or observations suggestive of the presence of the flag, is proposed in Figure 1. It is clear that while some factors need specialist input from therapist or psychologist, many factors can be addressed by rational and informed discussion with any health professional.

The psychosocial dimension: relevance for pain management

Psychosocial assessment can be left to professional psychology personnel in those clinics which have the luxury of these staff. Their absence from other clinics, however, does not mean that the task can be ignored. Psychological screening tests are available: though

- A for 'attitude'.
    'I am not getting up until this pain has gone'
    'This pain is my body's way of telling me to rest'
- B for 'behaviour'
    extended rest
    very high pain ratings (e.g. 11 on a 10-point scale)
    inappropriate use of walking aids/dark glasses, etc.
- C for 'compensation'
    the presence of ongoing litigation
    reliance on a benefit system for an income
- D for 'doctors'
    inappropriate and misleading information has been imparted:
        'The doctor told me I had a marshmallow spine'
        'They told me I would end up in a wheelchair'
- E for emotions
    depressed mood
- F for family
    family members excuse normal activity
- W for work
    there are severe physical stresses at work or job dissatisfaction

Figure 1: The Psychosocial 'Yellow Flags'.

designed for specialist psychological assessment by trained professionals, some of them are easily administered by the non-specialist. Most take the form of multiple-choice-type questions which can be completed by the patient in the clinic. Their value in the clinic that does not have psychological support is three-fold:

- They may help to identify the patient whose psychological scores are well outside the norm for the population and may thus be unsuitable for the limited expertise available in the clinic.
- They allow progress to be charted.
- They allow colleagues to share information using a common language.

On the other hand, there is evidence that the tests are not diagnostic on their own, and their use in quantifying the response to psychological treatments is disappointing.

In considering the psychosocial aspect, it is important for the clinician to distinguish between the multidimensional model and the concept of malingering. The presence of a degree of distress or illness behaviour is not indicative of malingering. It is not a sign of abnormal psychological function, even though some of its more idiosyncratic manifestations may cause wonder and, occasionally, amusement. Illness behaviour is a normal part of the experience of chronic pain.

Subjective experience of pain

The nociceptive system for pain has, at the interface between the individual and the environment, nerve endings of simple structure whose physiological activity varies according to the local environment. The type of word used tells us something about the subjective experience of pain and its effect on the individual. The McGill scoring system offers a choice of words to describe the pain. Some of them (like 'aching' or 'burning') are straightforward symptoms suggesting nociceptive or neuropathic pain. Others ('torturing' or 'agonizing') imply a degree of central nervous system integration of inputs.

Suffering and distress

Depressive thoughts and loss of self-esteem, even suicidal thoughts, are to be expected in a chronically painful condition. The premorbid state is relevant. In view of the common neurotransmitters involved in regulating mood and pain experience, there is good reason to view chronic pain and depression as diseases with features in common. There are several self-rating questionnaires which were developed for use in screening for depression but which have been successfully adapted for the chronic pain population. The hospital anxiety and depression index (HAD) and the modified Zung index are examples. 'Catastrophizing' is a technical term for 'fearing the worst' and refers to such emotions associated with thoughts such as 'I can't go on' or 'this pain is never going to get better'. It can, as part of a detailed psychological evaluation, be assessed in a quantitative way. 'Locus of control' is the technical term for the patient's view of the responsibility for pain management. The patient who looks to the professional for a cure is 'externally controlled', the one who is prepared to consider responsibility for self-management is 'internally controlled'.

Expectations and beliefs

The traditional medical model explains the purpose of pain in that pain has a protective function, promoting rest of the injured part, and warning of environmental hazards. This is a belief that persists when someone suffers chronic pain after an injury. This belief is an important determinant of persistent disability. It is influenced by the way in which the injury is managed by the attending professionals. For example, someone to whom the word 'arthritis' is synonymous with a wheelchair-bound parent will be reluctant to exercise the spine that has been described to have 'arthritic changes'. Similarly, the inevitable and appropriate caution with which an ambulance paramedic and a hospital doctor treat a road accident victim with neck pain or the patient with angina may lead to a state of hypervigilance in which very minor symptoms assume great significance, long after the nociceptive causes for the pain have resolved. This is known as 'symptom expectation'. The belief that there is an ongoing nociceptive cause and a continuing disease is an important determinant of chronicity. This belief can be perpetuated by the professional adopting a purely biomedical view of the symptoms, such as continuing to look for a cause of the pain. Requests for 'scans' to find a cause for the pain are common, and compliance with these requests may reinforce the patient's view that there is a serious problem. Repeated radiological examination may occasionally be useful in demonstrating to the patient that there has been no progressive damage, but the clinician must make sure that the patient understands the purpose of the examination. In particular, it is worth noting that if a patient expects that a test will show an abnormality, a normal result may worsen the patient's distress.

Complaints and non-verbal communication

Illness behaviour is the way in which a sufferer communicates the experience of pain. In its most easily observed form, this can take the form of grimacing or complaint on examination. The display of such behaviour is not governed entirely by the activity of nociceptors, but is influenced by cultural and social factors. Thus the frequency of reports of chronic neck pain after vehicle trauma may not correlate with the frequency of crashes in a particular country, but may be influenced by factors such as the availability of affordable health care, the number of professionals available to treat the condition and the ease of access to the litigation process. Simple clinical tools have the potential for producing illness behaviour, by drawing the sufferer's attention to the persistence of the condition. For example, keeping a diary of daily pain symptoms may lead to an inappropriate focusing on the persistence of these symptoms, a phenomenon known as 'symptom amplification'. Some patients wear cervical or lumbar supports in a way that makes their presence very visible, and they become 'fashion accessories'. Transcutaneous nerve stimulators can easily be concealed under clothing, but some patients wear them in a way in which they can easily be seen – for example in the breast pocket. Even drugs have the potential for allowing illness behaviour to be demonstrated: the transdermal preparations of opioids or glyceryl trinitrate can be worn under clothing, but may be worn prominently on exposed skin. Even a bottle of analgesic tablets may be carried prominently in a jacket pocket. The presence of illness behaviour is sometimes taken as 'evidence' that the patient is consciously exaggerating the symptoms for personal gain. This is an oversimplification that causes distress and leads to the adoption of an attitude to the patient that is not conducive to a therapeutic relationship. A number of factors govern the display of illness behaviour. In general terms, illness behaviour will persist (be reinforced) as long as attention to the behaviour is made, and may disappear (be extinguished) if attention is not forthcoming. The professional may be unable to influence the way in which behaviour will be reinforced or extinguished in the patient's day-to-day life, unless an attempt is made to involve family members.

The social environment

Management of the chronic pain patient involves rehabilitating the patient back into a meaningful role in society. This may require a careful assessment of the work and social environment, so that activity, when it is resumed, is undertaken at a level compatible with ability. The financial factor is significant amongst social influences. The patient who stands to lose all financial benefits if he manages to overcome the powerful demotivating influences of cognitive, affective and behavioural complications of chronic pain may fall at the last hurdle unless this issue is addressed.

Further reading

Ferrari R, Russell AS. Epidemiology of whiplash: an international dilemma. Annals of the Rheumatic Diseases 1999; 58: 1–5.

Kendal NAS, Linton SJ, Main CJ. Guide to assessing psychosocial yellow flags in acute low back pain: risk factors for long-term disability and work loss. Wellington, New Zealand: 1997. Accident Rehabilitation and Compensation Insurance Corporation of New Zealand and the National Health Committee, Ministry of Health, 1997; 1–22.

Related topics of interest

Back pain – medical management (p. 34); Depression and pain (p. 69); Psychosocial management of pain (p. 186).

PSYCHOSOCIAL MANAGEMENT OF PAIN

The aim of psychological management is one of changing the perception of sufferers, so that rather than considering themselves to be suffering from chronic illness, they consider themselves to be well and coping, and responsible for the maintenance of their own health.

The psychological management of pain addresses those features of the chronic pain syndrome described as cognitive and behavioural features. It does not attempt to provide relief from pain, although relief of pain is sometimes recorded as a result of treatment. Psychological management is sometimes deferred until all possible medical treatments have been concluded. This approach has the advantage that the sufferer cannot approach psychological treatments with an ambivalent attitude and has to accept that there is no medical cure for the pain. However, this particular approach has two problems. First, successive attempts to treat pain symptoms without addressing the psychosocial dimension risks making the distress worse with every failed intervention. Secondly, the approach engenders in the minds of all involved an unnecessary distinction, a dualism, between the medical cause and the psychosocial presentation. It has been suggested that psychosocial features are of relevance to the outcome of painful conditions within a short time of initial presentation, and that early intervention might prevent progression to a chronic pain syndrome.

Interview and self-rating questionnaires may describe the sufferer in terms of affective, cognitive, behavioural or functional impairment. Individualized treatment plans can be designed. An efficient use of resources is a Pain Management Programme which provides psychological management within a group setting. An advantage of this approach is the peer pressure that can be applied on members of the group. Programmes are typically outpatient activities, but inpatient programmes are suitable for isolated areas or where the patients are most disabled. The precise subject matter of programmes varies with the skill-mix and interest of the staff, but in general terms the treatment is termed cognitive behavioural therapy. An outline of the treatment of cognitive behavioural therapy is as follows, and is 'taught' or 'practised' within the context of a course of group instruction over a period of weeks or months.

Information

An explanation of the nature of chronic pain is necessary to overcome fears that pain is a sign of harm that requires rest. The concept of chronic pain as a disease as distinct from a symptom is difficult to grasp. Inadequate explanations or the unguarded use of medical jargon may have resulted in false beliefs about the presence of progressive disease. Inadequate understanding of the nature and purpose of investigations and treatment lead the pain sufferer to expect further tests or surgery. It is helpful to have an explanation from an expert about the limitations of medical treatment. Explanations about the role of analgesics, in particular about the hazards of using a 'pain contingent' or 'as required' dosing strategy, are also useful.

Coping skills

Strategies for dealing with exacerbations of pain can be introduced. The gate control theory of pain modulation can be used as a model to explain that many factors influence the perception of pain. Distraction techniques encourage the use of intensive mental or pleasurable activity, including relaxation techniques, to overcome the pain experience. Distraction techniques encourage the patient to develop an 'internal' way of managing distress, rather than relying on 'external' factors, such as analgesics or the physical attentions of a partner or health professional.

Mood modification

The effect of mood on the pain experience can be addressed by encouraging patients to challenge negative thoughts which accompany disability or an exacerbation of pain.

Activity modification

Inappropriate expectations of ability and fear of activity are features of the pain experience that need specific attention. The two concepts introduced are goal setting and pacing. Goal setting refers to a target for physical activity that is agreed between patient and professional, and pacing is the tactic by which this target is achieved. In the case of the patient who undertakes excess activity when pain is controlled and is then disabled by pain as a consequence of this activity, paced activity demands a disciplined approach to rest breaks and exercise. Activity goals during a programme are agreed by mutual consent: the patient is encouraged to start activity at a level compatible with pre-existing fitness and to increase this level progressively.

Behaviour modification

The psychological management of pain addresses those behaviours that cause the sufferer to become dependent on others. The overprotective partner is encouraged to allow the pain sufferer to undertake activities, and needs education about all the issues outlined above. Pain behaviour can be a threat to normal social functioning. It can be reduced by responses which pay little attention to the behaviour. This approach sees pain behaviours as responses that have been reinforced by inappropriate attention, such as encouragement to rest, continued investigation to find non-existent pathology and continued attempts to cure the pain.

Outcomes of cognitive behavioural therapy

Notwithstanding the difficulty in designing appropriate clinical trials comparing cognitive behavioural therapy with 'standard' treatment, there seems to be good evidence for efficacy in a number of different chronic pain conditions. A recent systematic review has reviewed 25 controlled trials. In these trials control groups remained on waiting lists or received basic medical, family or physiotherapy support. It is possible that many such control patients concomitantly received therapy from other therapists not included in the trial teams. The review examined outcomes studied by the trials in the reporting of pain experience, mood, coping strategies, activity levels and overt pain behaviour. In addition some trials examined the impact of cognitive behavioural therapy on fitness, social role functioning and use of health care system, including drug use. The review concluded that outcomes in many of these criteria were improved where cognitive behavioural therapy was included. In practical terms there is evidence to support cognitive behavioural therapy for conditions including low back pain, irritable bowel syndrome and conditions in which pain may be associated, such as the chronic fatigue syndrome.

Systematic reviews

Evans G, Richards S. Low back pain: an evaluation of therapeutic interventions. University of Bristol, Health Care Evaluation Unit, 1996; 176.
Morley S, Eccleston C, Williams A. Systematic review and meta-analysis of randomised controlled trials of cognitive behaviour therapy and behaviour therapy for chronic pain in adults, excluding headache. Pain 1999; 80: 1–13.

Related topics of interest

Back pain – medical management (p. 34); Irritable bowel and oesophageal pain (p. 89); Musculoskeletal pain syndromes (p. 95); Psychosocial assessment (p. 181).

SPECIAL CIRCUMSTANCES – CHILDREN

Pain in children has historically been underestimated, and consequently undertreated. There are fundamental differences in the perception of pain, and the response to therapeutic interventions, from the adult population.

Paediatrics represents a continuum of physical change. Important considerations include:

- In the nervous system, the basic neurological structures required to perceive pain are developed at around 26 weeks. This is when the thalamocortical fibres penetrate the cortical plate. Responses to stimuli are seen as early as 7 weeks' gestation.
- In the neonate, water represents 80% of total body weight, with a markedly reduced percentage of muscle and fat. This leads to a proportionately increased volume of distribution for water-soluble drugs, but reduced active sites for binding, leading to increased plasma levels.
- There is an increased cardiac output, leading to rapid equilibration of drug levels, and an immature blood–brain barrier, allowing for a relatively larger amount of water-soluble drugs entering the central nervous system (CNS).
- The importance of providing comprehensive analgesia and anaesthesia to infants is vital in preventing damaging changes in physiological and behavioural responses to painful stimuli. Failure to provide analgesia is ethically unjustified. Clear demonstrations of changes in the neuroendocrine axis, and more recently responses of the brain under functional magnetic resonance imaging (fMRI), has resigned the practice of providing muscle relaxation with minimal sedation or pain relief to history.

Assessment

0–3 years. This is the most difficult period for the health care professional. Crucial factors to take into account are the underlying cause of the pain (diagnosis, operation, etc.), the current status of analgesic treatments and behavioural measures. In practice, the behavioural factors are the opinion of parents or other carers who know the child and can recognize the difference between a cry of pain, of hunger or of frustration. Physiological measures (heart rate, blood pressure, SaO_2) have some statistical use, but are rarely helpful in the clinical scenario.

>3 years. The use of a variety of 'Pain Rating Scales' adapted for use in children are valuable. The most widely known are the pictures of faces, from happy to crying, and the use of 'poker chips' to represent 'pieces of hurt'. Pitfalls can occur if the mode of analgesic support (e.g. intramuscular injection) creates a greater level of distress than the pain. Again, behavioural assessment may be the only tool available, or may supplement the self-assessment measures. Specialist staff and time with the children are important in explaining how the systems work, and may need to be considered in the preoperative period.

Treatment

The main issues dealt with here will be the use of medicines; however, it must not be forgotten that, as with adults, heightened anxiety can increase any pain, and the level of pharmacological intervention may be reduced by the presence of family, the distraction of play and specially trained staff.

The principles of the World Health Organization (WHO) analgesic ladder are valuable, as is regular assessment to avoid recurrence of pain at the end of a dose, and modes of administration that do not frighten the child.

Paracetamol is a widely used, safe analgesic in all age groups. It can be administered orally, rectally and intravenously. Where possible, the oral route is to be preferred, but in the very young or if there is gastrointestinal upset, the parenteral routes can be used. Intravenous administration, of course, requires the presence of an intravenous cannula, something that may itself frighten.

Nonsteroidal anti-inflammatory drugs (NSAIDs) should be considered early in the management of paediatric pain. Ibuprofen and diclofenac are both licensed for use in children in the UK. Both may be used orally, but diclofenac is also available in a rectal formulation. Dosing is calculated by means of lean body mass, with modifiers for age. Aspirin is no longer used as a result of a rare, but potentially fatal liver complication, Reye's syndrome.

Opioids may be valuable. Codeine and morphine are the drugs most widely used. The intramuscular route is best avoided, and the use of indwelling subcutaneous cannulae is complicated by variable absorption, and the real, if lesser, discomfort of injection.

Up to 1 year, infusions of morphine may be used but the risks of apnoea and convulsions are significant, and appropriate supervision or respiratory support is necessary. The pharmacokinetics of morphine are similar to those in adults by about 1 year; prior to this, increased half-life and consequent increase in plasma levels must be considered with infusions or repeated intermittent dosing. From 1 to 4 years old, oral supplementation with either codeine or morphine may be appropriate when the need is low, and infusions may be appropriate. Another technique uses a nurse as a 'proxy' to activate the mechanism of a patient-controlled analgesia (PCA) device. This technique, which bypasses one of the intrinsic safety barriers to PCA, requires training of staff and advice to relatives. After 5 years old, most children can be taught how to use a PCA device. Good preoperative education is important.

Regional anaesthesia. Single-shot caudal epidurals are widely used for surgery involving sacral to mid-thoracic dermatomal involvement. In infants and young children, the caudal route may be used to insert catheters to the lumbar or even thoracic region. The spinal cord extends to about L3 at birth, reaching its adult level of around L1 by the end of the first year, and this needs to be taken into account if neuroaxial techniques are being considered. As the importance of analgesia in children is recognized, there is now more widespread use of regional techniques. It is important to discuss these with the child, as the unfamiliar sensation of numbness may be distressing if it is (to the child) unexpectedly present in the postoperative period.

Chronic pain

Children suffer from chronic pain. Various surveys have suggested an incidence of 5–10%. This may vary from the obvious pain relating to a disease process, e.g. juvenile rheumatoid arthritis, with both chronic and acute components, to more complex pain problems in which psychosocial issues (family, friends, school, etc.) play a crucial role.

Assessment

Assessment must also encompass the developmental changes which have a profound effect on cognition, behaviour and the biological status of the child, and which are undergoing constant change.

Core aspects of the pain to be elucidated are:

- Developmental level.
- What degree of understanding does the child, and family, have of the pain.
- Medical history – especially conditions in which pain is a component of the disease or its treatment.
- Affect and behaviour of the child and any evidence of previous problems.
- Social – how pain affects the family, schooling and peer groups.
- Management – what mechanisms do the child use in different spheres of life to cope with the pain.

In the preverbal child, most of the assessment tools have been developed for acute pain. Principal areas of research have concentrated on facial expressions, crying and behavioural scales. However, these may prove misleading as the ability to express different aspects of a distressing situation are limited by the developmental stage of the child, and, in the very young, it may not be possible to differentiate chronic pain from any other chronic symptom.

Once language skills begin to be acquired, as in adults, there are a number of questionnaire tools available, and more dependence can be placed on the responses of the child, without relying wholly on a parent or carer.

Treatment

As in adults, there is a wide spectrum of conditions, and treatments will vary from the relatively simple medication and interventional approaches to more inclusive multidisciplinary requirements.

Neuropathic pain conditions are seen in children, most commonly related to trauma, either accidental or surgical. Common diagnoses seen are:

- Peripheral nerve injuries.
- Post-amputation.
- Complex regional pain syndromes

Non-pharmacological methods must include time spent with the child, parent and siblings, to explain the nature of the problem in a language and environment they are comfortable with. As the child grows up, and the challenges of disability become more difficult within the peer groups, there will be increasing and differing needs from those at the onset of the condition.

The basic approach is similar to that used in adults (see appropriate chapters). This is essentially the cognitive behavioural approach adapted to the family context, and is an active area of research. Drug management in children is notoriously difficult because of the paucity of data. On an empirical basis, anticonvulsant drugs are more commonly licensed and evaluated in children from a safety point of view than antidepressant drugs, although a number of the tricyclic antidepressants are licensed for low-dose use in nocturnal enuresis.

Pain conditions in which the biopsychosocial model will need to be applied at an early stage include:

- Recurrent abdominal pain.
- Headaches.
- Chest pain.
- Non-specific limb pain.

In all such cases, as in adults, it is important to exclude serious pathology as early as possible, to reassure, to prevent the development of 'treatment-seeking' behaviours, and to develop a self-management system which has a reduced (or absent) need for direct health care services and as limited an effect as possible on social and educational development.

This does not exclude the need for drugs, injections, physiotherapy, etc., but places them in a framework that the child and family easily understand and accept to reduce time away from the normal activities of daily life.

Further reading

British National Formulary (BNF) for Children.

SPECIAL CIRCUMSTANCES – THE ELDERLY

The population of Western countries is ageing, which presents the clinician with special challenges. Specific painful conditions such as post-herpetic neuralgia and pain after stroke afflict the older population, whereas conditions such as osteoarthritis become increasingly important with advancing age. The older patient may be unable to communicate to health professionals because of deafness or cognitive decline, and prior experience of illness or privation (such as surviving a war) may lead to an attitude of stoicism, with unreported pain. The concept that older patients suffer less pain with advancing age is unfounded, unhelpful and results in undertreatment of pain.

Physiological changes of ageing

The nervous system

There is a progressive loss of neural tissue with age, and myelinated large fibres are more sensitive to age-related loss than small unmyelinated fibres. The effect of herpes zoster on the older population is believed in part to be due to this differential loss.

There is some evidence to suggest that sensory thresholds obtained during nerve stimulation (performed, for example, prior to nerve lesioning in the treatment of chronic pain) may increase with age. It is accepted, however, that there is an increase in sensitivity to mechanically induced pain with age.

There is evidence from animal studies of reductions in opioid receptor density and increases in receptor affinity, and an increase in pain sensitivity with increasing age.

Cognitive decline

Alzheimer's dementia is a disease in which the cortical functions responsible for processing sensory information become progressively impaired. This occurs in the presence of normal functioning of the somatosensory cortex. The implication from this is that sensory thresholds are not affected by the disease process and that pain continues to be experienced, although the expression and understanding associated with the sensation of pain is impaired.

Metabolism and drug handling

The major alterations in body composition with ageing are the reduction of body water, an increase in fat and a change in protein binding of drugs. The effect of such changes is a reduction in the volume of distribution (i.e. a higher initial plasma concentration for a given dose of drug). Age-related reductions of metabolism in the liver and clearance by the kidney are associated with higher concentrations of drug with continuous dosing: both transdermal fentanyl and oral dihydrocodeine have been shown to be affected by this.

Aspects of management

Management of acute pain requires accurate assessment of pain and the use of adequate doses of analgesics. The elderly hospitalized patient may present acutely with delirium or may have pre-existing cognitive decline that renders the simplest approach to pain assessment very difficult. Simple tools, such as visual analogue scales, or even questions about the intensity of pain may be poorly understood. Third-party opinions, for example from spouse or nursing home staff, may be valuable. Facial expressions and other behaviour may be used to assess the degree of pain.

Management of chronic pain is a rehabilitation exercise in which the patient's circumstances have to be considered. Independent living may be compromised by the sedative side effects of analgesic medication. Activities such as using kitchen equipment and driving are important factors in maintaining independence, and a drug with a sedative side effect that is responsible for a loss of confidence and ability to carry out such tasks, or worse still an accident, is of limited benefit. If the case for such medication is overwhelming, it is important that it is introduced in a way that the impact of such side effects is minimized: a mentally competent spouse or other family member living in the home clearly puts the patient at an advantage. In other cases, it may be appropriate to consider a change from independent living to one in which the patient is discretely supervised.

SPECIAL CIRCUMSTANCES – LEARNING DIFFICULTIES

People with intellectual disabilities are amongst the most disadvantaged in society in terms of satisfying their health care needs. Although significant advances have been made, there is still little research on the management of pain in people with learning difficulties. Cognitive impairment causes late presentation of illness, unreliable self-reporting of pain, difficulty in understanding pain and difficulties in decision-making and consent to treatment. Initial assessment and evaluation of therapy is difficult. Furthermore, those with cognitive impairment are at risk of more complex and severe illness and more likely to undergo painful surgical procedures. Quantitative somatosensory testing of pain threshold in individuals with mental retardation suggests than they are more sensitive to heat pain than normal people. Communication difficulties are a commonly cited reason for inadequate provision of health care, so it beholds the health care provider to improve communication methods. Communication through carers may mean that the accuracy of the history is lost. Assessment has been undertaken through physiological, behavioural and socioemotional responses depending on functional ability and level of disability.

Research shows children with severe cognitive impairment suffer pain frequently, mostly due to accidental injury, and children with the fewest abilities experience the most pain. These children rely on a willingness of carers to interpret behavioural and emotional manifestations as pain and an ability to understand them; research has shown that children with cognitive impairment receive smaller total opioid doses postoperative following spinal fusion surgery than those without cognitive impairment. Such discrepancy in pain management practice has to be eradicated.

Further research is needed to develop reliable and effective assessment tools.

SPINAL CORD INJURY

Pain is a common symptom in patients with spinal cord injuries and contributes significantly to the morbidity of the condition. In some studies, it has been the pain, rather than the paraplegia, which has been the reason for inability to work. Pain may be related to the disability or the injury.

Pathophysiology

The physiology of pain sensation after spinal cord injury has to explain the varied and distressing syndromes that are observed. The clinical picture may be confused by the presence of an incomplete lesion, or a second lesion at a lower segment of the cord.

Traditional neuroanatomy has described the effects of partial spinal cord section. Sensory changes are said to be dissociative. In the Brown-Séquard syndrome of partial cord section, selective modalities are lost because the spinothalamic pathway (temperature and pain) crosses the midline near the level of the spinal root and the dorsal column (proprioception and mechanoreceptor) does not. Similarly, the development of a syrinx, a cystic lesion within the spinal cord, is associated with characteristic sensory and motor changes. There is a loss of pain sensation due to destruction of fibres crossing over in the spinal cord, but light touch and positional sense is preserved.

Explanations based on gross anatomical findings do not, however, explain other phenomena. Central pain syndromes occur even in the absence of a spinal cord. They can be extraordinarily complicated in their presentation, with the patient 'experiencing' not only pain but also movement and related phenomena such as fatigue. Inhibition of modulating descending pathways accounts for some, but not all, of the increased activity of dorsal horn neurones immediately above the level of injury. In an animal experimental spinal cord preparation, abnormal activity in visceral afferents to non-noxious stimulation is due to this mechanism, and may be responsible for the exaggerated cardiovascular response that is seen with bladder distension and catheterization. Dorsal horn sensitization by nerve damage and continuing nociceptive stimulation may account for some of the changes.

Clinical features

The spinally injured patient may present with a complete or incomplete lesion. Careful evaluation will sometimes reveal a second lesion at a lower level of the cord than the primary lesion. This may be the site of specific symptoms that would confuse the unwary. There are thus many ways in which the spinally injured patient can present.

Nociceptive pain may be overlooked as a cause of pain, unless there is an obvious other injury to account for it. The assumption that nociceptive pain will not be experienced distal to a spinal cord lesion is a dangerous one, for it fails to consider the situation with an incomplete lesion, and the effect of central disinhibition of nerve pathways which enter the cord above the level of the lesion. The causes of nociceptive pain include:

- Soft tissue trauma.
- Spinal fractures.
- Mechanical instability of the spine.
- Osteoporotic vertebral collapse.
- Pressure areas.
- Overuse of upper limbs to compensate for disability.
- Painful muscle spasm.

Neuropathic pain presents as segmental pain at the level of injury, with an area of hyperalgesia at the boundary between normal and abnormal sensation. The level of lesion is rarely precise and subtle differences in modality loss may be detected for several segments above the clinical level of the lesion. Rarely, changes of a type I complex regional pain syndrome (CRPS I) may be apparent in the dermatomal distribution corresponding to the site of the lesion. In the case of an incomplete lesion, a root lesion at a lower level may be symptomatic.

Causes of neuropathic pain include:

- Spinal cord damage.
- Compression of nerve roots.
- Compression of spinal cord by bone fragments, haematoma and scar tissue.
- Syrinx development within the spinal cord.
- Changes within the brain itself (central pain).

Central pain is of insidious onset and may occur weeks to months after the injury. Central pain may have a visceral quality. It is experienced as a burning sensation below the level of the lesion, though poorly localized, and alterations of pain and temperature sensitivity (indicative of spinothalamic tract involvement) are noticed on examination.

Management

Treatment of pain after spinal injury requires accurate diagnosis as to the cause of the pain. Abdominal causes should be excluded before the pain is assumed to be of central origin. Visceral stimulation, either by abdominal pathology or physiological processes, is dangerous when the spinal cord injury has removed the inhibitory influence on spinal reflexes. It can lead to fatal hypertension or arrhythmias.

With the exception of selective destruction of the dorsal root entry zone (DREZ) lesion for intractable segmental pain, procedures to destroy nerves are inappropriate. Surgical removal of the diseased spinal cord may result in central pain, and less drastic destruction procedures prevent the patient taking advantage of future surgical advances. Spinal decompression and stabilization is appropriate in some cases, and prevents further injury to the cord. Counter-stimulation techniques – transcutaneous electrical nerve stimulation (TENS) and spinal cord stimulation (SCS) – can be used when dorsal column nerve tracts remain intact.

Patients with spinal cord injury may be taking many medications and it is difficult to establish what is the specific contribution of any particular drug. However, the scheme below offers a rationale for treatment, with the evidence available summarized:

- *Tricyclic antidepressants* are valuable in many neuropathic pain states and should be considered in the management of the neuropathic pain of spinal cord injury.
- *Anticonvulsants* are valuable in many neuropathic pain states and should be considered in the management of the neuropathic pain after spinal cord injury. Gabapentin has been shown to reduce spasticity and improve the quality of life of patients with spinal cord injury, at least when used in combination with other drugs.
- *Baclofen* has been shown to reduce painful spasticity. It can be administered by the intrathecal route.
- *Opioids*. They may be worth a therapeutic trial, and have been reported to be successful in some patients.

General and psychological support for the victim of spinal injury has a role to play in preventing the morbidity of chronic pain. Pain relief has in the past received relatively little attention, and the low frequency of reports of pain has been said to be due to patients and carers adopting a stoical attitude to an inexplicable and untreatable complication.

Related topics of interest

Anatomy and physiology (p. 5); Multiple sclerosis (p. 91); Stroke (p. 199).

STROKE

A number of mechanisms may be responsible for the pain experienced by the victim of a stroke. Associated neurological impairment may make it difficult for pain relief to be obtained by changing position, and expressive difficulty may result in the patient suffering silently. Interpretation of complaints may be made more difficult by the emotional lability and depression encountered in some patients. Although the term 'thalamic pain' referring to a specific lesion in the central nervous system (CNS) was first used in 1906, it is clear that lesions in any part of the central nervous system can result in neuropathic pain. The term central post-stroke pain (CPSP) is therefore more appropriate. However it is also very important to realize that stroke victims also experience nociceptive pain as a consequence of postural abnormalities, spasm, contractures and pressure areas, and it may be premature to conclude an automatic diagnosis of CPSP just because of the history of stroke. Pain arising from these other causes needs specific treatment.

Central post-stroke pain

Pathology

Any lesion of the CNS can be implicated as the cause of central pain. No single area has to be involved and there are no patterns of symptoms pertaining to any particular lesion. Pain can be experienced after haemorrhagic or thrombotic/embolic stroke. Loss of afferent input causes neuronal hyperpolarization and increased burst firing. Hyperpolarization of neurones normally involved in nociception signals the sensation of pain. Abnormal burst firing is influenced by the activity of several neurotransmitters including serotonin, noradrenaline, glutamate, γ-amino butyric acid (GABA) and histamine.

Clinical features

There are many features, and the diagnosis cannnot be confirmed from the description alone. Most commonly it is described as burning, aching, lancinating, pricking, lacerating or pressing. There may be a background of pain which is constant or intermittent with added paroxysms of pain. It can be deep or superficial or both. It may be localized, for example to the hand or even only one side of the hand, or it may cover large areas such as the whole of the right or left side or the lower half of the body. Patients find it relatively easy to define the extent of the area of their pain. The development of pain cannot be prevented. It may occur immediately or be noticed only several months after the stroke. Autonomic changes may also be noticed. Concomitant depression or distress may compound the presentation. The diagnosis of CPSP has as a prerequisite the presence of a partial sensory loss. Allodynia and hyperalgesia also define the syndrome, being present in up to 75% of sufferers, but are not essential for its diagnosis.

Management

Alternative diagnosis should be sought and excluded. Examples are the common phenomenon of shoulder pain that affects up to 25% of patients within 2 weeks, and pains related to posture, spasticity or immobility. With the proviso that these conditions, which may lend themselves to simple specific mobilization procedures or alterations to nursing routine, have been excluded, the following drugs and techniques may have a place in management:

Antidepressants. A single controlled study has estimated the NNT (number needed to treat) for antidepressants for pain after stroke to be 1.7. These drugs are thus considered first-line treatments. There is precedent from other studies of neuropathic pain for using the tricyclic antidepressants, but there is some evidence to support the use of clomipramine as opposed to nortriptyline. In the population, predominantly elderly, under consideration, however, the anticholinergic actions of tricyclic drugs such as amitriptyline may have undesirable side effects on cognitive functioning.

Anticonvulsants. Sodium valproate, phenytoin and carbamazepine have been claimed to be of benefit, but the latter has not withstood the scrutiny of controlled trial. Gabapentin, a drug that has been shown to be of benefit in painful spasticity in multiple sclerosis, has been used with effect in post-stroke pain.

Antiarrhythmic drugs. Patients who have failed to respond to adrenergic tricyclic antidepressant drugs have been reported to respond to mexiletine.

Other treatments variously described include oral ketamine, transcutaneous nerve stimulation and spinal cord stimulation. A further development of stimulation technique is motor cortex stimulation, in which electrodes are implanted during craniotomy. This has been reported to be of value in some face and shoulder pains following stroke. Attempts to improve circulatory abnormalities with sympathectomy or vasodilators such as nifedipine have also been reported.

Postural abnormalities and spasm

Shoulder pain may result from glenohumeral subluxation, and strategies designed to improve the range of movement and function of the glenohumeral joint may be valuable. These may include surface electrical stimulation, which has been shown to improve the range of passive lateral rotation of the humerus. Some patients may develop refractory pain and movement limitation for which more vigorous attempts at passive mobilization are required. Botulinum toxin has been reported of value for the relief of spasm. The overall rehabilitation of the patient, however, including the psychological well-being, is important in managing the pain. Strategies for positioning and movement taught by a physiotherapist with experience in the field may obviate the need for drug treatment. Local anaesthetic block may provide short-term relief of pain and spasm and allow active and passive movement around joints to be undertaken.

Further reading

Jensen TS, Lenz FA. Central post-stroke pain: a challenge for the scientist and clinician. Pain 1995; 61: 161–4.

Related topics of interest

Neuromodulation – TENS, acupuncture and laser photobiomodulation (p. 146); Spinal cord injury (p. 196); Therapy – antidepressants (p. 209); Therapy – ketamine and other NMDA antagonists (p. 221).

SYMPATHETIC NERVOUS SYSTEM AND PAIN

Peripheral nociceptor activity causes an increase in efferent sympathetic discharge, but under normal circumstances, sympathetic activity has no impact on the discharge of nociceptive neurones.

Although there is some debate as to the usefulness of such a distinction, when nociceptors appear to be under the influence of the sympathetic nervous system, pain is described as sympathetically maintained pain (SMP). When nociception is unaffected by the sympathetic nervous system, the pain is described as sympathetically independent pain (SIP). The sympathetic nervous system may be involved in pain at any part of the neuraxis. Sympathetic nerve blocks may affect pain if it has a sympathetic component. Noradrenergically, active drugs applied to the periphery, the spinal cord or centrally, affect pain, which has a sympathetic component. Some neuropathic pain and some cases of complex regional pain syndromes (CRPS) are sympathetically maintained. CRPS has signs directly associated with the sympathetic nervous system and is a more complex clinical picture than simply a sympathetically maintained neuropathic pain.

Mechanisms

The mechanisms for pain which responds to sympathetic nerve blockade are:

- Peripheral nociceptors which are sensitive to noradrenaline.
- Sympathetic efferent activity producing low-grade ongoing activity in nociceptors.
- Sprouting of sympathetic nerve fibres in dorsal root ganglia.
- The stimulation of α receptors in the dorsal horn.
- The altered levels of centrally acting monoamines.

Diagnosis

A diagnosis of SMP is made by response to various manipulations of the sympathetic nervous system.

The intravenous phentolamine test. Phentolamine is an α_1 and α_2 adrenergic antagonist. It prevents excitation of noradrenaline-sensitive nociceptors. Phentolamine in normal saline (30 mg 100 ml^{-1}) is infused over 20 min. If pain is relieved, it is believed that the pain is sympathetically maintained.

Sympathetic local anaesthetic blocks by preventing efferent sympathetic activity also allow an assessment of the place of the sympathetic nervous system in the maintenance of the pain. Although local anaesthetics preferentially block preganglionic sympathetic fibres, false-positive results can be produced by blocking nociceptive afferents but sensory testing will alert to this.

Intravenous regional sympathetic blockade using a guanethidine tourniquet technique helps diagnosis. Guanethidine in normal saline (10–20 mg/ 20–50 ml) is injected into a limb which has been exsanguinated and to which a tourniquet has been applied. Dilution of guanethidine in a prilocaine solution enhances patient comfort during the procedure.

Sympathomimetic drugs. SMP can be provoked by sympathomimetic drugs.

Treatments

Intravenous regional sympathetic blockade. This technique is widely used for the treatment of sympathetically maintained pain. It comprises the injection of guanethidine to an exsanguinated limb, isolated by a tourniquet. Systematic review has failed to show difference in the treatment of CRPS between guanethidine and placebo. Despite this conclusion, and the suggestion leading from this, that the technique is of little value, intravenous guanethidine sympathetic block is commonly performed, and its use is believed to be justified by the past success of uncontrolled trials. It is suggested that the technique may work as a consequence of the tourniquet, causing differential nerve blockade as a result of pressure and ischaemia. Guanethidine displaces noradrenaline from nerve endings. When it is used in intravenous regional sympathetic blockade, pain can transiently worsen as displacement initially increases circulating amounts of noradrenaline. Allodynia has been demonstrated during the block. The worsening of pain and the allodynia can be protected against by adding prilocaine to guanethidine for injection. Guanethidine is also available in tablet form.

Clonidine. Clonidine is an α_2 adrenergic agonist. Experimentally and clinically it has been shown to have an antinociceptive effect. It is effective in treating SMP. The understanding of its mechanism suggests a further role in the treatment of noradrenaline-sensitive neuromata.

Clonidine has a spinal and supraspinal action. It inhibits the release of noradrenaline from primary afferents both in the dorsal horn and at higher centres. This is a presynaptic α_2 action. Clonidine also effects cholinergic transmission and inhibits acetylcholinesterase.

Clonidine is available as an oral preparation, and used at doses of 50–150 µg t.d.s. The absence of neurotoxicity allows intrathecal and epidural use. Used in this way it is valuable for the treatment of cancer pain when opioids are ineffective or the patient is troubled by side effects of opioids.

Consistent with the mechanism of its main use, the treatment of hypertension, clonidine causes hypotension. Rebound hypertension can occur if treatment is suddenly stopped. Bradycardia occurs. Sedation, anticholinergic effects and respiratory depression can occur.

Tizanidine has an α_2 agonist action. It is used mainly for its antispastic (useful in stump jactitation) effects but may be useful where a myofascial and neuropathic process coexist. Dose recommendations are 2–24 mg daily in 3–4 divided doses. It does however have very sedating effects and may be best taken as a single night-time dose.

Adrenergic β-antagonists. Propranolol, a β_2 antagonist, has been reported effective in phantom limb pain and painful diabetic neuropathy.

Neuroleptic drugs. These work through post-synaptic α blockade. Although their use is not common, they have been reported to be of use as single preparations and in combination with amitriptyline.

Further reading

Dickenson E. Spinal cord pharmacology of pain. British Journal of Anaesthesia 1995; 75: 193–200.

Glynn C, Dawson D, Sanders R. A double-blind comparison between epidural morphine and epidural clonidine in patients with chronic non-cancer pain. Pain 1988; 34: 123–8.

Systematic review

Jadad AR, Carroll D, Glynn CJ, McQuay HJ. Intravenous regional sympathetic blockade for pain relief in reflex sympathetic dystrophy: a systematic review and a randomised, double-blind crossover study. Journal of Pain and Symptom Management 1995; 10(1): 13–20.

Related topics of interest

Anatomy and physiology (p. 5); Cancer pain – drugs (p. 50).

THERAPY – ANTIARRHYTHMICS

The constant barrages of afferent fibre activity that characterize neuropathic pain states depend on influx and efflux of sodium ions through axonal membrane sodium channels. Some anticonvulsants and some antiarrhythmics block sodium channels and give relief from some neuropathic pain. Anticonvulsants are considered in their own chapter.

The antiarrhythmics most commonly considered are intravenous or transdermal lidocaine and mexiletine.

Lidocaine

Lidocaine has been shown to be effective in peripheral nerve damage, post-herpetic neuralgia and painful diabetic neuropathy, but not in cancer-related pain. The best documented effective dose was 5 mg kg^{-1}, and when infused over 30 min was well tolerated. Adverse effects of lightheadedness and nausea and the possibility of cardiac arrhythmias must be considered. Lidocaine should not be used in patients taking other antiarrhythmics, and tricyclic antidepressants should be stopped.

The longer-term effects of intravenous lidocaine have not been considered, although one randomized controlled trial noted a significant effect lasting up to 8 days. There is no evidence for the longer-term efficacy or safety.

Intranasal lidocaine (20–80 mg) has been shown to provide significantly better pain relief than saline.

Open-label trials have found a lidocaine 5% patch to be effective in the treatment of post-herpetic neuralgia. The patch is applied for 12 out of 24 hours and a 6-week treatment period is recommended. Absorption is minimal, with up to four patches worn for 24 hours. The most common adverse effect is skin irritation at the site of application.

Mexiletine

There is no evidence for the commonly held belief that response to intravenous lidocaine is predictive of response to mexiletine. Oral mexiletine 750 mg daily was effective in two out of four randomized controlled trials. It has also been shown to be effective in HIV-induced peripheral neuropathy.

Two trials have shown it to be effective in painful diabetic neuropathy, but another study shows it to have a number needed to treat (NNT) of 10.

Pain due to peripheral nerve damage is said to respond, but pain due to spinal cord injury is said not to respond.

At moderate doses for neuropathic pain, 675 mg daily, up to 50% of patients developed side effects of nausea, vomiting, abdominal pain, dizziness, headache and tremor.

Mexilitine should be started at 100–200 mg daily in divided doses and increased slowly.

Systematic review

Kalso E, Tramer MR, McQuay HJ, Moore RA. Systemic local anaesthetic type drugs in chronic pain: a systematic review. European Journal of Pain 1998; 2: 3–14.

Related topics of interest

Anatomy and physiology (p. 5); Therapy – anticonvulsants (p. 207).

THERAPY – ANTICONVULSANTS

The constant barrages of afferent fibre activity that characterize neuropathic pain states depend on influx and efflux of sodium ions through axonal membrane sodium channels. Drugs which block sodium channels can give relief from some neuropathic pains. Sodium channels are blocked by some anticonvulsants.

The mainstays of pharmacological treatment of neuropathic pain are the antidepressants and the anticonvulsants. Conventionally, the anticonvulsants remain second-line treatment for neuropathic pain. Pharmacological methods may help but rarely are completely successful. A multidisciplinary approach to non-pharmacological and behavioural methods is required. Evidence from randomized controlled trials supports the use of anticonvulsants in painful diabetic neuropathy (PDN) and post-herpetic neuralgia (PHN). The effects on specific features of neuropathic pain, namely allodynia and hyperalgesia, have been used as indicators of efficacy. Neuropathic pain syndromes may present with various clinical subtypes, depending on the severity of the nerve injury and the extent to which the central nervous system has become sensitized. Subtypes can be described with reference to the effectiveness of different therapies in the condition. Anticonvulsants act by membrane stabilization. Although empirical advice, based on the pathophysiology described above, has traditionally been that anticonvulsants are first-line treatment for 'lancinating' or 'stabbing' features of neuropathic pain, conventionally they remain second-line treatments after antidepressants. Significant differences between the efficacy of gabapentin and amitriptyline have not been demonstrated. Anticonvulsants are useful in combination with tricyclic antidepressants to spare increases in dose and consequent side effects. A systematic review of the use of anticonvulsants for diabetic neuropathy and post-herpetic neuralgia offered no evidence that gabapentin is any better then other anticonvulsants.

Carbamazepine has been shown to relieve pain of trigeminal neuralgia to maximum doses of 600–2040 mg/day and given for 5–14 days. In doses of 600 mg/day for 2 weeks it has been shown to reduce the pain of diabetic neuropathy. It is started at a low dose 100 mg once to twice a day; a common dose is 200 mg three to four times a day.

Phenytoin 300 mg/day for 2 weeks has been shown to be effective in PDN. Unwanted troublesome side effects are common with carbamazepine and phenytoin. Carbamazepine and phenytoin are licensed for use in trigeminal neuralgia.

Lamotrigine has been shown to relieve trigeminal neuralgia when titrated to 400 mg/day over 4 days. It has also been shown to relieve the pain of peripheral neuropathy secondary to HIV when titrated slowly to 300 mg/day. Rash is relatively common and more severe skin reactions can occur but tend to be at inappropriately high doses. Dose titration to an effective level needs to be undertaken cautiously.

Topiramate has been shown to be effective in PDN, starting at a dose of 25 mg o.d. increasing to 200 mg twice a day over a 2-week period. Its effectiveness is also claimed in mixed neuropathic pain, in which pain was improved at a mean dose of 214 mg/day (weekly titration of 25–50 mg is suggested), post-thoracotomy pain at a dose of 50 mg in the morning and 75 mg at night, and trigeminal neuralgia secondary to multiple sclerosis at a dose of 150 mg/day. Fatigue and weight loss are significant side effects.

Gabapentin has an unknown mechanism of action. Its effectiveness has been demonstrated in randomized controlled trials of PDN and PHN. Both pain and its physical consequences such as sleep disturbance were improved. The number needed to treat (NNT) for gabapentin is 3.2 for PHN and 3.7 for PDN. Effectiveness is claimed for the treatment of neuropathic pain in trigeminal neuralgia, complex regional pain syndromes, multiple sclerosis, neuropathic cancer pain and neuropathic back pain. The dose recommendations are to reach a range of 0.9–1.8 g/day by a daily dose increase of 300 mg. Dose escalation can be problematic and limited by side effects of drowsiness and dizziness (in up to 25%). Ataxia, a more disabling side effect, can be a problem, but gabapentin has fewer toxic effects than carbamazepine and phenytoin. It has no known drug interactions. Gabapentin is licensed for the treatment of neuropathic pain of any cause. Recent work also suggests that it is able to improve the quality of pain relief after surgery, and reduces the requirement for epidural analgesia.

Pregabalin is licensed for the management of peripheral neuropathic pain. Pregabalin, S-isobutyl-γ-amino butyric acid (GABA), binds to the $\alpha_2\delta$ subunit of voltage-gated calcium channels on presynaptic nerve terminals and modulates calcium influx into the cell. This reduces the excessive release of excitatory neurotransmitters such as glutamate, noradrenaline and substance P, which is a mechanism of neuropathic pain.

There have been 10 randomized double-blind, placebo-controlled studies of pregabalin's use in neuropathic pain: 5 in PDN and 4 in PHN and 1 in both conditions.

In PHN, pregabalin was effective in relieving neuropathic pain in 3 out of the 4 studies. At 150, 300 and 600 mg/day compared with placebo it was statistically significant in relieving pain. The NNT for decreases in pain scores of >30% was 2.7 and for decreases of >50% was 3.4.

In PDN, pregabalin was effective in relieving neuropathic pain in 4 out of 5 studies. At 300 and 600 mg/day it was statistically effective compared with placebo.

Dizziness and somnolence were the most frequent adverse events, resulting in discontinuation in 10.8% of the pregabalin group compared with 5% of the placebo group.

The recommended dosing schedule is 75 mg twice a day for 3–7 days, then 150 mg twice a day for 1 week, increasing to 300 mg twice a day as indicated.

Systematic reviews

Collins SL, Moore RA, McQuay HJ, Wiffen P. Antidepressants and anticonvulsants for diabetic neuropathy and post-herpetic neuralgia: a quantitative systematic review. Journal of Pain and Symptom Management 2000; 20(6): 449–58.

McQuay H, Carroll D, Jadad AR, Wiffen P, Moore A. Anticonvulsant drugs for management of pain: a systematic review. British Medical Journal 1995; 311: 1047–52.

Wiffen P, Collins S, McQuay H, et al. Anticonvulsant drugs for acute and chronic pain (Cochrane review). In: the Cochrane Library, Issue 3, 2000, Oxford, Update software.

Related topic of interest

Therapy – antidepressants (p. 209).

THERAPY – ANTIDEPRESSANTS

The mainstays of pharmacological treatment of neuropathic pain are the antidepressants and the anticonvulsants. These drugs alleviate pain but do not treat the whole pain problem. A multidisciplinary approach to non-pharmacological and behavioural methods may be required.

A systematic review of 21 studies, looking at 10 different antidepressants in several painful syndromes showed 30% of patients will have >50% pain relief. The overall number needed to treat (NNT) is 2.9, with NNT of 2.4 for painful diabetic neuropathy, 2.3 for post-herpetic neuralgia and 2.5 for peripheral nerve injury and central pain. Although all types of antidepressants have been suggested for use in the treatment of neuropathic pain, tricyclic drugs are more efficient than heterocyclic drugs. There is no evidence that any one tricyclic drug is better than another but side effects may influence choice. Thus nortriptyline is frequently preferred to amitriptyline because it has less anticholinergic effects, such as dry mouth, sedation and constipation.

Analgesic effect has been shown to be independent of the effect on mood. However additional benefit may be accrued from the effect of antidepressants on the reactive component of pain. There is evidence that patients with a substantial physical basis for their back pain responded to desipramine as well as patients who did not have a physical basis. In addition it has been shown that:

- Analgesic effect is not significantly different for pain with an organic or psychological basis.
- Analgesic effect is not significantly different in the presence or absence of depression.
- Analgesic effect is not significantly different in doses smaller than those usually effective in treating depression and in normal doses.
- Antidepressants which inhibit monoamines less selectively are more effective than selective drugs, indicating that noradrenaline and serotonin are both involved in the mechanism of pain.

The role of antidepressants in the management of low back pain is controversial: on the one hand, pain relief is not consistently obtained; on the other hand, associated symptoms and functional ability may be improved.

Tricyclic antidepressants

The commonly used tricyclic antidepressants (TCAs) are nortriptyline, amitriptyline, dosulepin and imipramine. Analgesic response occurs much faster (within 4 days) than antidepressant response. TCAs prevent the reuptake of endogenous noradrenaline and serotonin. Serotonin and noradrenaline within the central nervous system (CNS) enhance the action of the descending inhibitory neural pathways at spinal cord level. To spare anticholinergic side effects such as drowsiness and dry mouth, small doses of nortriptyline and amitriptyline such as 10 mg at night in the elderly or 25 mg at night in the more robust or imipramine 25–50 mg twice a day are used. Patients should be encouraged that side effects reduce over time. As side effects allow, dose can be increased at weekly intervals to achieve further therapeutic effect. Sedating antidepressants should be considered if there are problems of sleep disturbance.

Selective serotonin reuptake inhibitors

Selective serotonin reuptake inhibitors (SSRIs) have been demonstrated to work in the treatment of chronic pain, but research and experience of them is limited. Paroxetine 40 mg daily has been used to treat painful diabetic neuropathy; however, systematic review suggests NNT for paroxetine of 6.7, which compares unfavourably with the demonstrated efficacy of a substantial dose of imipramine with NNT of 1.4 and other TCAs at 2.4. Paroxetine and mianserin have been shown to be less effective than impipramine in various painful conditions.

Notwithstanding the comments made above about efficacy, fluoxetine and paroxetine have been shown to have a lower incidence of side effects than TCAs. They may have a role where the tricyclics cannot be tolerated. A systematic review recommends non-selective antidepressants to be used for depressed patients with pain complaints if antidepressants are a suitable treatment for the depression, for patients with pain of organic basis where other treatments have failed and for patients with chronic pain in the head region. It is important for the sake of the patient's self-confidence and the relationship with the doctor that the patient is aware he has been prescribed an antidepressant, albeit for a different indication.

The role of the newer groups of antidepressants in chronic pain has not been established.

Systematic reviews

McQuay HJ, Tramer M, Nye BA, et al. A systematic review of antidepressants in neuropathic pain. Pain 1996; 68: 217–27.

Onghena P, Van Houdenhove B. Antidepressant-induced analgesia in chronic non-malignant pain: a meta-analysis of 39 placebo-controlled studies. Pain 1992; 49(2): 205–19.

Volmink J, Lancaster T, Gray S, Silagy C. Treatments for postherpetic neuralgia – a systematic review of randomized controlled trials. Family Practitioner 1996; 13: 84–91.

Related topics of interest

Depression and pain (p. 69); Neuralgia – post herpetic (p. 131).

THERAPY – ANTI-INFLAMMATORY DRUGS

There are two principal types of medication to be reviewed: the non-specific nonsteroidal anti-inflammatory drugs (NSAIDs) and the cyclo-oxygenase type 2 inhibitors (COXIBs). They both act through the inhibition of the cyclo-oxygenase enzyme, thereby preventing the synthesis of prostaglandin, a precursor to a number of other inflammatory mediators. From the pain perspective their crucial role is in the sensitization of primary afferent nociceptors. Cyclo-oxygenase is recognized as existing in at least two isoenzymes. The type 1 or constitutive enzyme, is involved particularly in platelet function, preserving the integrity of the gastric mucosal barrier and in regulating renal tubular blood flow. The type 2, or inducible enzyme, is the principal mediator in pain, but is also present in vascular endothelium and renal tissue.

Non-selective inhibition of both isoenzymes is a feature of the NSAIDs and relatively specific inhibition of the type 2 (inducible) enzyme is a feature of the COXIBs.

Uses and efficacy: acute pain

Many NSAIDs have been trialled in a standard acute pain model (e.g. following dental extraction), and found to be effective. The number needed to treat (NNT) for single doses is well established in controlled trials: diclofenac 50 mg, NNT = 2.3; ibuprofen 400 mg, NNT = 2.4.

In the context of more traumatic surgery, the following factors need to be considered:

- The question of alternate routes of administration for patients for whom the oral route is excluded (e.g. starved for surgery, postoperative gastric motility problems, etc.). There are rectal and parenteral formulations of several NSAIDs and one parenteral COXIB.
- The issue of platelet function inhibition, and the risk of bleeding due to surgery or trauma.
- The risk of renal dysfunction, particularly in patients in whom hypovolaemia is difficult to manage, or with pre-existing renal disease.

Topical NSAIDs have been shown to be effective for musculoskeletal pain syndromes: acute syndromes (measured at 7 days), NNT = 3.8; chronic syndromes (measured at 14 days), NNT = 4.4.

NSAIDs and COXIBs are usefully considered as agents whose use may allow a reduction of other drugs, including opioids, rather than agents that have to be used.

Use and efficacy: chronic pain

Choice of drugs is influenced by the side-effect profile, and the drugs should be used at the lowest effective dose and for the shortest period of time. The *British National Formulary (BNF)* classifies the gastrointestinal risk of NSAIDs into highest (azathioprine), intermediate (e.g. diclofenac, naproxen) and lowest (ibuprofen).

Ibuprofen used at doses of 200–800 mg three times daily has a 5–15% incidence of gastric side effects, which makes it a reasonable first choice. Gastric protection with a proton pump inhibitor or misoprostol should be considered. Compound preparations of the latter with NSAIDs are available, but are absolutely contraindicated in pregnancy, and relatively contraindicated in women of childbearing age. The decision to use COXIBs is subject to the guidelines discussed below. The use of NSAIDs for the routine management of musculoskeletal pain is popular, but, in the absence of an acute inflammatory process, controversial. Consideration must be made of the long-term risks. The action of NSAIDs on the pain processing systems of the spinal cord may explain why these drugs remain popular with patients and are reported to be of benefit even in the absence of inflammation.

COXIB controversy

It has long been recognized that a significant morbidity and mortality of the 'non-selective' drugs was due to inhibition of the type 1 isoenzyme, leading to loss of gastroprotective effects and the risk of gastrointestinal bleeding. The mortality in some patient groups is as high as 18%. Other problems were increased bleeding due to altered platelet function (especially in the perioperative period), and renal problems, ranging from mild peripheral oedema, to hypertension, to acute and chronic renal failure.

Studies with the COXIBs confirmed the anticipated absence of effect on platelet adhesion and improved gastrointestinal morbidity and mortality. However, hypertension and peripheral oedema were noted. Four drugs initially came to market in the UK: rofecoxib, celecoxib, etoricoxib and valdecoxib.

Two large clinical trials confirmed the advantages of selective cyclo-oxygenase inhibition on gastrointestinal safety. VIGOR, the **Vi**oxx **G**astrointestinal **O**utcomes **R**esearch, found a lower incidence of gastrointestinal complications in patients taking rofecoxib compared with naproxen. The study was performed on patients with rheumatoid arthritis who were not allowed to take aspirin (aspirin being a non-specific cyclooxygenase inhibitor). CLASS, the **C**elecoxib **L**ong-term **A**rthritis **S**afety **S**tudy, compared celecoxib with ibuprofen or diclofenac. It allowed the use of aspirin where indicated. Both trials confirmed the superior gastrointestinal profile of the COXIBs, but more importantly the overall mortality was noted to be higher in the rofecoxib arm of the VIGOR study. The CLASS trial showed no significant mortality difference between the NSAIDs and the COXIBs. A further US trial on the effect of rofecoxib versus placebo on the incidence of bowel cancer was halted after concerns of increased mortality in the rofecoxib arm. The increase in mortality was due to an increase in cardiovascular and cerebrovascular events The drug was voluntarily withdrawn from the market soon after. A systematic review of 14 controlled trials of celecoxib described an eightfold reduction in the incidence of gastrointestinal ulcer complications with the use of celecoxib compared with non-selective NSAIDs, and no evidence of increased mortality. The increased risk appears to be due to a combination of renal dysfunction, leading to hypertension and fluid retention, and the unopposed action of isoenzyme 1 activity in platelets and the vascular endothelium. This had been initially noted during the VIGOR trial, but its significance had been overlooked because both rheumatoid arthritis and non-use of aspirin were themselves risk factors for vascular disease. The future with respect to COXIBs is unclear, with two of the four COXIBs having been withdrawn from the market and a fifth having had its application process suspended. There is still a need for an anti-inflammatory drug free of adverse gastrointestinal effects, but there is a requirement to balance this with due caution over long-term cardiovascular safety.

In the United Kingdom, the National Institute for Clinical Excellence (NICE) initially published guidelines restricting the use of COXIBs in arthritis to certain groups of patients, specifically elderly patients believed to be at risk of gastrointestinal adverse effects and those requiring long-term maintenance on high-dose NSAIDs. This guidance was superseded after the withdrawal of rofecoxib.

The UK Committee on Safety of Medicines has recommended that COXIBs are not used in patients with known cardiovascular or cerebrovascular disease, and that in respect of both NSAIDs and COXIBs, the lowest dose is used for the shortest time necessary.

Non-selective inhibition: further concerns

Recent attention has focused on the cardiovascular safety of the 'non-selective' NSAIDs. Aspirin has long been used due to its ability to provide non-reversible inhibition of cyclo-oxygenase in platelets, and so reduce cardiovascular-related mortality. However all the other 'non-selective' NSAIDs provide reversible inhibition, and although perioperative bleeding due to platelet dysfunction continues to be an issue, it is unclear whether other factors relating to these drugs may be leading to an increased cardiovascular mortality.

Further reading

British National Formulary.

THERAPY – BOTULINUM TOXIN

Botulinum toxin is licensed for the symptomatic treatment of blepharospasm and hemi-facial spasm. It is used without licence to relieve pains due to other types of muscle spasm.

The pharmaceutical preparation contains botulinum toxin of the type A serotype, serum albumin and sodium chloride. The botulinum toxin was first isolated in 1895 from the food of victims of food poisoning. It was then first recognized as a neurotoxin.

Mechanism

The neurotoxic action reduces neuromuscular transmission, thereby causing skeletal muscle weakness and inhibition of muscle spasm. Botulinum toxin selectively acts on peripheral cholinergic nerve endings. It enters the nerve terminal and causes localized chemical destruction. This prevents the release of acetylcholine at the neuromuscular junction. Efficient neuromuscular transmission depends on the release of acetylcholine from the axonal terminal and its binding to the postsynaptic receptors to effect the muscle action potential. Without the synthesis and release of acetylcholine the muscle action potential is prevented. After the nerve end plate has shrivelled, it starts to regenerate by sprouting. When the sprouts reach the muscle surface a new neuromuscular junction has formed. Regeneration takes approximately 3 months. When it is complete, tone and muscle spasms recur. At that stage the injection of botulinum toxin can be repeated indefinitely. Tachyphylaxis has been shown. In addition to its effects on the motor nerve ending, botulinum toxin has also been reported to have an analgesic effect.

Pharmacokinetics

Botulinum toxin is given intramuscularly to affected peripheral muscles. Its spread is dependent on the dose of drug and the volume of diluent. It is taken up by neuronal transport to the spinal cord where it is broken down to inactive metabolites.

Use

Botulinum toxin is available in single-patient-use vials each containing 100 units. The preparation is freeze dried. It is recommended that it be reconstituted with normal saline, although workers in the USA are using local anaesthetic as solvent to enhance the speed of onset of effect. Diluted with normal saline, the toxin's onset of action is at approximately 3 days and the effect peaks at 1–2 weeks after administration. Injections are sometimes carried out under electromyographic control or with the use of radio-opaque dye and fluoroscopy.

The manufacturer's recommended maximum dose in the treatment of blepharospasm is 100 units per 12 weeks. The maximum dose used by workers in the USA for the relief of other muscle spasms is 400 units per 12 weeks.

The LD_{50} for single use in a 70 kg person is 3000 units. Depending on the size and number of muscles needing treatment, doses as small as 1.25 units are used for blepharospasm and 30 units for painful conditions secondary to muscle spasm. Inhibition of muscle activity of 50% allows the performance of otherwise difficult physiotherapy. The physiotherapy brings further improvement in muscle function. Painful conditions in which botulinum toxin has been used include:

- Back and myofascial pain.
- Spasticity and painful contractures.
- Headache.

There is evidence of efficacy in all these conditions, but systematic reviews on the use of botulinum in spasticity do not comment specifically on pain control.

Back and myofascial pains. Botulinum has been shown to be effective in low back pain when injected paravertebrally at five sites, 40 units per site. Botulinum toxin has been used to treat myofascial pains of the neck, shoulder and low back. Injections have also been carried out to psoas and quadratus lumborum muscles to relieve spasticity. Muscle spasm precipitating pain in conditions such as multiple sclerosis has been treated. Pain caused by an abnormal posture forced by muscle spasm can be treated by botulinum toxin.

Spasticity and painful contractures. Secondary contractures resulting from neurological deficit after stroke or from disuse, as in the complex regional pain syndromes (CRPS), is reported to be relieved by botulinum toxin. In cervical dystonia over 70% have pain. The injection of doses of botulinum toxin ranging from 100 to 236 units has been reported to give relief of spasm with consequent reduction in pain. In all these conditions the relief of spasticity offers an opportunity and is not an alternative to this.

Headache. Botulinum has been shown to be effective in the prevention of tension headache and migraine.

Side effects

Local muscle weakness can occur from local spread of drug. Injections into the neck may thus affect swallowing. Misplaced injections can paralyse nearby muscle groups extensively. Excessive doses may paralyse muscles distant to the site of injection. Spread is affected by both dose and volume of diluent. Generalized malaise, about which the patient should be informed, can follow the treatment.

Botulinum toxin is potent in reducing muscle spasm and, although currently unlicensed for the purpose, there may be a place for it in the relief of muscle spasm which causes pain. It has been found to have few side effects. The established regeneration of nerve makes it acceptable in terms of no long-term destructive effect. It offers a useful addition to the pain clinician's armamentarium as a drug which may relieve pain and also improve function.

Further reading

Childers MK, Wilson DJ, Galate JF, Smith BK. Treatment of painful muscle syndromes with botulinum toxin: a review. Journal of Back and Musculoskeletal Rehabilitation 1998; 10(2): 89–96.

Racz G. Botulinum as a new approach for refractory pain syndromes. Pain Digest 1998; 8(6): 353–6.

Raj PP. Botulinum for the treatment of pain (editorial). Pain Digest 1998; 8(6): 335–6.

Systematic review

Ade Hall RA, Moore AP. Botulinum toxin type A in the treatment of lower limb spasticity in cerebral palsy. In: the Cochrane Library, Issue 4, 2000. Oxford: Update software.

Related topics of interest

Complex regional pain syndromes (p. 60); Multiple sclerosis (p. 91).

THERAPY – CANNABINOIDS

The cannabinoids are derived from the resin of the plant *Cannabis sativa*. The only known active constituent is 9-tetrahydrocannabinol (δ9–THC). Other cannabinoids are an oral synthetic nitrogen analogue of THC and intramuscular levonantradol. There are claims for their use in nausea and vomiting, appetite stimulation in HIV-infected patients, movement disorders and glaucoma. There have also been claims that cannabinoids are useful in the treatment of migraine and painful spasticity in multiple sclerosis and spinal cord injury. There is some evidence that they are analgesic in humans. A systematic review of nine randomized controlled trials has concluded that there need to be further trials into their use in spasticity and neuropathic pain but they have no place in the management of postoperative pain. A double-blind comparison with placebo in a patient with prior history of cannabinoid use has demonstrated an opioid-sparing effect in chronic pain.

Mechanisms of action

It is suggested from animal studies that cannabinoids reduce the behaviour believed to equate with the clinical syndromes of allodynia and hyperalgesia. From animal evidence, here summarized, it is believed that the brain is probably the site of action, but there is evidence for a spinal cord site of action.

Opioid receptor agonism. Perinatal exposure to cannabinoids results in analgesia, morphine tolerance and an abstinence syndrome when given naloxone. Naloxone and other opioid receptor antagonists, specifically the κ_1 antagonists, block the antinociceptive actions of cannabinoids. They do not prevent the behavioural effects. An effect has been observed when the opioid receptor is blocked by spinal administration.

Cannabinoid receptor agonism. Cannabinoid receptors have been identified; CB1 receptors on central and peripheral neurons and CB2 receptors on immune cells. The identification and cloning of specific cannabinoid receptors has been followed by the identification of an endogenous ligand called anandamide. The function of these receptors and ligands remains unclear. Cannabinoid receptor activation reduces the amplitude of voltage-gated calcium currents, thereby decreasing excitability and neurotransmitter release. The finding of further subclasses of receptors offers potential for separating analgesic actions from the harmful psychotropic actions by the development of synthetic analogues. The spleen contains cannabinoid receptors.

Prostaglandin metabolism. Anandamide is an intermediate product of arachidonic acid metabolism. Synthetic cannabinoids have been shown to reduce arachidonic acid-induced inflammation, presumably by an action on inhibition of eicosanoid synthesis.

Pharmacokinetics

δ9-THC is highly lipid-soluble and readily absorbed from the gastrointestinal tract and lungs. Bioavailability after oral ingestion is about 6%. It has, like other lipid-soluble compounds, a large volume of distribution. It is metabolized to polar water-soluble compounds before excretion by the kidney, although intestinal elimination accounts for some of the drug.

Clinical effects

The best that can be achieved with cannabis is an antinociceptive effect equivalent to 60 mg codeine. The anti-inflammatory effect is unlikely to be as valuable as the currently available drugs. There is inadequate evidence to support their use in the management of more complex pain. In addition to the actions described above, cannabinoids lower intraocular pressure. Inhalation of the drug is associated with carboxyhaemoglobin production, and intrauterine growth retardation and an increase in childhood leukaemia are features of the children of women who use cannabinoids in pregnancy. Central nervous system side effects include psychomotor and cognitive impairment. Psychiatric syndromes encountered with cannabinoid use include mania, anxiety and depression, and there is a six-fold greater incidence of schizophrenia in heavy users than in non-users.

Any potential clinical benefit in the management of chronic pain must be weighed against the hazards of the drug, and the potential harm that may result from widespread availability and social acceptability if legalization were undertaken.

Systematic review

Campbell FA, Tramer MR, Carroll D, et al. Are cannabinoids an effective and safe treatment option in the management of pain? A qualitative systematic review. British Medical Journal 2001; 323: 13–16.

Further reading

Doyle E, Spence AA. Cannabis as a medicine? British Journal of Anaesthesia 1995; 74: 359–61.
Holdcroft A, Smith M, Jacklin A, et al. Pain relief with oral cannabinoids in familial Mediterranean fever. Anaesthesia 1997; 52: 483–6.
Robson P. Cannabis as a medicine: time for the phoenix to rise? British Medical Journal 1998; 316: 1034–5.

Related topic of interest

Multiple sclerosis (p. 91).

THERAPY – CAPSAICIN

Capsaicin is a specific chemical entity, 8-methyl-*N*-vanillyl-nonenamide, of the capsaicinoid family. Capsaicinoids are molecules derived from chilli peppers. Capsaicin, which is formulated as a single drug for the treatment of neuropathic pain at 0.075% concentration and musculoskeletal pain at 0.025% concentration, is also found in a variety of compound rubefacients sold in pharmacies and other retail outlets.

Mechanism of action

There is a specific receptor for capsaicinoids called VR1. It is present only on a subpopulation of C fibres. These fibres, as well as generating pain, are involved in a process known as neurogenic inflammation. This is a phenomenon mediated via nerve growth factors and other chemical messengers carried within microtubular structures of the nerve and responsible for a localized anti-inflammatory response. After initial exposure, the neurones become insensitive to all other stimuli including further capsaicin. This requires that capsaicin is regularly applied to desensitize the nerve and deplete transmitters. It also works by depletion of substance P from the C-fibre endings in the periphery and the dorsal horn.

Efficacy

Neuropathic pain. A recent systematic review calculated a number needed to treat (NNT) of 5.7 at 8 weeks for a variety of neuropathic pains. Taken as individual conditions the data, from smaller-sized trials, support the use of capsaicin: painful diabetic neuropathy, NNT = 5.9; post-herpetic neuralgia, NNT = 5.3; peripheral nerve injury, NNT = 3.5.

Musculoskeletal pain. The use of 0.025% capsaicin over 8 weeks has been studied with a systematic review of controlled trials. This has commented on the wide variation in reporting of success with trials, but calculates NNT of 8.1. More specific syndromes might respond more readily; thus, 3 trials calculate NNT of 3.3 over 4 weeks for osteoarthritis of the knee.

In addition, benefit is claimed for neuropathic stump pain, neck pain, loin pain – haematuria syndrome, complex regional pain syndromes (CRPS) and cutaneous pain associated with tumour. Intranasal application has been reported effective in cluster headaches.

Very high concentrations of 5–10% have been used in CRPS and neuropathic pain. The irritant effect of such high concentrations requires that the drug is administered under regional blockade. One technique involves the application of the concentrated preparation into the ureters after catheterization at cystoscopy: epidural analgesia is required for several days.

Capsaicin is being studied for the treatment of cystitis, pain associated with human immunodeficiency virus and painful or itching cutaneous disorders from scars.

Adverse effects

There were no serious adverse effects reported during a study looking at application for an average of 20 weeks. Stinging and burning at the application site occurs in 59% of patients but this was mainly in the first week and disappeared over the course of the study, consistent with its mechanism of action. There are anecdotal reports of attenuation of stinging and burning by the application of a local anaesthetic preparation before the capsaicin.

Systematic review

Mason L, Moore RA, Derry S, Edwards JE, McQuay HJ. Systematic review of topical capsaicin for the treatment of chronic pain. British Medical Journal 2004; 328: 991–4.

Related topic of interest

Anatomy and physiology (p. 5).

THERAPY – KETAMINE AND OTHER NMDA ANTAGONISTS

Ketamine is an anaesthetic drug with a few notable features which have resulted in its introduction to pain clinic practice. The rationale for its use is supported by animal studies which allow tentative conclusions to be drawn about a mechanism of action. However, the extrapolation of animal data, based on electrophysiological and behavioural studies, to the human experience of pain is always difficult. The evidence to support the use of ketamine in chronic pain is necessarily limited. Ketamine is valuable for its excellent analgesic properties at subanaesthetic doses, and at anaesthetic doses for its freedom from the effects of cardiovascular and pharyngeal reflex depression which characterize other anaesthetic agents. As such it has a unique place for providing analgesia and anaesthesia for environments in which other agents would be difficult to use: for example at the site of a major accident or on the battlefield. The drug is limited by major side effects, however: notably cardiovascular stimulation, increased cerebral blood flow, and psychological disturbance. The role of the NMDA system and 'windup' in the production of a chronic pain syndrome has not been clearly elucidated. It has been shown however that subanaesthetic doses of i.v. ketamine of 0.5 mg kg^{-1} bolus followed by 0.25 mg kg^{-1} h^{-1} reduce hyperalgesia and are an adjuvant in postoperative analgesia.

Mechanisms of action

The animal experimental evidence for a mechanism of action includes the following:

N-methyl-D-aspartate receptor (NMDA) antagonism. NMDA receptors are believed to be involved in the spinal cord processing of nociceptive input, where they respond to excitatory amino acids released from the central processes of primary afferent nociceptors. Their activation by nociceptors is believed to result in a response, 'windup', which may outlast the duration of action of the activation impulse and stimulate the spinal cord cell to metabolic activity. Their inactivation by ketamine is suggested, but not proven, as a manoeuvre to prevent the development of a chronic pain syndrome. It is further suggested that the observed synergism between opioids and ketamine is mediated via a common action on the NMDA receptor. In animal models of neuropathic pain, ketamine appears to restore opioid responsiveness.

Opioid receptor agonism. Binding of ketamine to opioid receptors in central nervous system tissue has been observed.

Serotoninergic and adrenergic mechanisms. Synaptic uptake of serotonin and noradrenaline is inhibited, and the antinociceptive action of spinally administered ketamine can be reversed by phentolamine and serotonin receptor antagonists.

Cholinergic mechanisms. Physostigmine, a centrally acting anticholinesterase, can reverse the sedation and anaesthesia of ketamine, while 4-aminopyridine, an antagonist of competitive neuromuscular blockade, speeds recovery from ketamine anaesthesia.

Pharmacokinetics

Ketamine is metabolized in the liver to an active metabolite, norketamine, which has analgesic properties, but is believed to have fewer side effects than ketamine. In this respect, oral treatment, despite a bioavailability of only 17%, may be preferred over parenteral treatment, where the benefits of the active metabolite are not obtained.

Pharmacodynamics

The incidence and severity of the two major side effects are dose related. Cardiovascular side effects include increases in heart rate, blood pressure, cardiac output, systemic vascular resistance and pulmonary artery pressure, and can be attenuated by benzodiazepines. Their origin is in the stimulation of the central nervous system by the drug, and because of this, the drug is contra-indicated in the presence of raised intracranial pressure or seizures. The psychological disturbances take the form of alterations of mood or body image, feelings of spatial disorientation, vivid dreams, hallucinations, pleasant or unpleasant illusions and complicated emergence from anaesthesia. They can occur with the use of ketamine by infusion for analgesia. Their occurrence can be reduced by the use of slow infusion rates. Intravenous midazolam is effective in countering the side effects observed after intravenous ketamine. This is used at doses between 2.5 and 15 mg per day, as an infusion. Alternatives are the use of oral midazolam, 0.5 mg kg^{-1}, or diazepam 5–10 mg. Haloperidol 2–4 mg is an alternative.

Clinical uses

Ketamine is used in malignant and non-malignant neuropathic pain. No oral preparation is available; the parenteral preparation is given orally or sublingually. A suggested oral dose is 50 mg and sublingually 10 mg, both three times a day. The dose can be titrated against response and side effects.

Ketamine has been shown to reduce pain in fibromyalgia. For cancer pain, ketamine has been used for incident pain, painful cutaneous lesions, bone pain, tenesmus and neuropathic pain, including the pain of spinal cord compression. Its use is best considered as an alternative or adjunct to opioids where they are ineffective or poorly tolerated. Subcutaneous and intravenous infusions at rates of between 40 and 500 mg per 24 hours have given relief: there is a wide variation in response which requires the titration of drug to achieve a response. The subcutaneous route is complicated by the presence of a skin reaction in 20% of patients, which requires regular resiting of the subcutaneous cannula.

Severe phantom limb pain and post-herpetic neuralgia have been reported to respond to parenteral ketamine. The single dose for intravenous response is reported between 0.125 and 0.3 mg kg^{-1}, or as an infusion at 0.2 mg kg^{-1} h^{-1}.

Ketamine is available in a preservative-free form for epidural and intrathecal use but this should be undertaken with caution. Ketamine administered epidurally has been reported as being effective in the treatment of complex regional pain syndrome type 1.

Other *N*-methyl D-aspartate receptor antagonists

Worldwide, the clinically available NMDA antagonists are ketamine, dextromethorphan, memantine, amantadine and three clinically used opioids which have NMDA activity, methadone, dextropropoxyphene and ketobemidone. There are reports of the success of all of these in modulating pain and hyperalgesia.

Further reading

Idvall J. Ketamine, a review of clinical applications. Anaesthetic Pharmacology Review 1995; 3: 82–9.

Luczak J, Dickenson AH, Kotlinska-Lemieszek A. The role of ketamine, an NMDA receptor antagonist, in the management of pain. Progress in Palliative Care 1995; 3: 127–34.

Mercadante S. Ketamine in cancer pain: an update. Palliative Medicine 1996; 10: 225–30.

Related topics of interest

Anatomy and physiology (p. 5); Cancer pain – drugs (p. 50).

THERAPY – OPIOIDS IN CHRONIC PAIN

Opioids are our most powerful analgesics, but politics, prejudice and our continuing ignorance still impede optimum prescribing. What happens when opioids are given to someone in pain is different from what happens when they are given to someone not in pain. The medical use of opioids does not create drug addicts, and restrictions on this medical use hurt patients.

Professor Henry McQuay
*University of Oxfor*d

Opioids are an acceptable mainstay for treatment of acute pain and moderate to severe cancer pain. Acute pain is usually nociceptive, transmitted by normal pathways and responds predictably to monotherapy over a limited time course. Patients with chronic pain often have ill-defined pathology, with complex biological, psychological and social dimensions. When treating postoperative pain or pain due to cancer, alleviating symptoms is the main goal, whereas in the management of chronic non-cancer pain the goal is not only relief of pain but also to keep the patient functioning, physically, socially and mentally. The treatment of chronic non-cancer pain with opioids remains controversial. However there is an ever-increasing consensus that some patients with chronic pain respond well to opioids when used in an overall rehabilitation plan.

The British Pain Society published its recommendations for the appropriate use of opioids for persistent non-cancer pain in 2004. They are based on evidence of effectiveness in the treatment of chronic non-cancer pain, but acknowledge there is a lack of data in many areas such as long-term efficacy and adverse effects where advice is based on clinical experience. They provide a balanced framework in which pain specialists and primary care doctors can make more informed decisions in partnership with patients. It is hoped that working within the framework will protect patients from adverse effects of opioid therapy, ensure careful follow up and define circumstances in which treatment will be stopped.

One of the aims of the recommendations is to discuss the well-documented problems of undertreatment, fuelled by concerns about patients' behaviour, tolerance, dependence and addiction which cannot be studied in randomized and placebo-controlled studies. The emphasis is that opioids should always be used in the context of an integrated rehabilitation plan that aims to improve physical and social function.

The recommendations, while emphasizing the importance of specialist teams, acknowledge that access to these services is limited. This may mean that primary care physicians have to take responsibility for patient care and analgesic prescribing while they await referral. Therefore close working relationships and good communication are needed between primary and secondary care services involving management of patients on opioids.

Clinical pharmacology

The analgesic action of opioids is mediated via receptors in the central nervous system. Three types of receptors are involved in the analgesia of opioids: these are the μ, κ and δ receptors. Receptors are identified in the brain, the spinal cord and afferent neurones. Receptor sensitivity may be enhanced by an inflammatory process and reduced by neuropathic pain mechanisms. Some of the action of opioid drugs may be mediated indirectly via an action on adrenergic and serotoninergic modulation of the spinal cord. Presynaptic action on the primary afferent C fibre is believed to be an important site of action. Morphine, local anaesthetic, ketamine and nonsteroidal anti-inflammatory drugs (NSAIDs) may have synergistic actions in preventing the process of neuronal sensitization.

All clinically useful opioids are μ agonists, but use has been made of partial agonists such as buprenorphine and nalbuphine. Buprenorphine is a partial μ agonist, and nalbuphine a partial κ agonist which has antagonistic actions at the μ receptor. Tramadol is a μ, κ and δ agonist which stimulates the release of serotonin and inhibits the reuptake of noradrenaline. It is useful to consider opioids as weak or strong depending on their relative efficacy. Codeine is a weak opioid, whose effects are maximum at about 200 mg per day. Strong opioids include morphine, its prodrug diamorphine, fentanyl, oxycodone, hydromorphone, methadone and buprenorphine. Transdermal preparations of fentanyl and buprenorphine are now available and marketing authorization has been given for their use in non-cancer pain. If one opioid is not effective, an alternative may be tried. The practice of 'opioid rotation', pioneered in the management of cancer pain, is worth trying in chronic non-cancer pain. The logic of this technique, in which different opioids are used to maintain analgesia while minimizing side effects, is attributed to incomplete cross-tolerance between different opioids.

Side effects

The effects of opioids when used for acute control of the nociceptive pain of injury are well known and include respiratory depression, sedation, nausea and pupillary constriction. However, in the context of the chronic pain sufferer, these physiological events are of less importance than the issues of dependency, tolerance and addiction, which are considered in detail below.

Nausea, vomiting, itching and somnolence are common and usually occur during the first few days of treatment. In the majority of patients these decrease with time. Constipation occurs in approximately 90% of patients receiving opioids; laxatives (stimulant and stool softening) should be routinely prescribed for all patients taking opioids unless there is a clear contraindication. Cognitive effects are common when treatment is started or doses changed; this may affect ability to drive, but research suggests patients who have reached a stable dose are generally fit to drive. Patients planning pregnancy should be warned of the possible effects on neonatal well-being (50% risk of withdrawal symptoms in newborn babies of mothers on opioid therapy), but risks should be balanced with benefits to the mother.

Recent views are that myoclonus and disturbing dreams are symptoms of opioid toxicity. Long-term use is linked with immunosuppression and endocrine dysfunction in <1% of patients. This may manifest as loss of libido, sexual dysfunction, irregular menses, galactorrhoea and reduced adrenal function. This latter condition, if suspected, requires urgent investigation by an appropriate specialist.

Opioid dependency, tolerance and addiction

These three terms are used interchangeably in error to describe the effect of reduction of clinical effect with duration of treatment, and lead to incorrect assumptions about the value of treatment and incorrect judgement about the behaviour of the patient. It is therefore useful to distinguish between the terms.

Dependence is an adaptive state to the presence of a drug manifest by intense physical disturbance (abstinence syndrome) when the drug is withdrawn. Initially described in volunteers without pain, and in subjects who have a history of recreational drug use, it remains poorly understood in chronic pain sufferers. It is said that patients who are denied opioids following successful treatment of a painful condition develop some features of this abstinence syndrome but that it is very different from that which occurs when subjects accustomed to recreational opioids are denied them. Physiological changes of opioid withdrawal include gastrointestinal disturbance, restlessness and perspiration. In the recreational user the symptoms are more dramatic and associated with a craving for drug and drug-seeking behaviour. The claims that specific opioids are to be preferred because of an intrinsic safety due to lack of 'dependency potential' have to be judged in the light of the poor understanding we have of dependency in the chronic pain sufferer. More accurately, it is the route of administration and the effect of variations of drug concentrations that may influence a tendency to dependency. Water-soluble drugs are more easily injected into the body, whereas lipid-soluble drugs achieve a rapid effect on the central nervous system. Rapidly rising drug concentrations in the dopamine pathways of the mesolimbic system and the periaqueductal grey cells lead to an increase in dopaminergic activity, and this activity may promote behaviour to acquire more of the drug.

Tolerance is the diminution of effect of drug with time, or the need to increase dose to maintain an effect. Tolerance is considered as a normal and expected response and not of harmful significance. In observing the opioid requirement of the patient with a static disease process, tolerance results in the progressive reduction of effect and the need for an increased dose. It is said that there is a ceiling for tolerance and that, once this is reached, further demands for increase have to be explained in other ways, such as worsening pathology, psychological distress or depression or the unmasking of a tendency to addiction. Tolerance extends the usefulness of the drug, since tolerance to side effects also occurs. Tolerance is a result of several mechanisms, of which the following are notable:

- A pharmocokinetic action, such as the induction of enzymes, or the accumulation of metabolites with antagonist properties (e.g. morphine-3-glucuronide).
- A pharmacodynamic action that results from changes in the drug receptor.

Addiction is a term reserved for the behaviour associated with the compulsive use of drugs, without regard for the clinical indication, and despite harm. It can conveniently be considered a brain disease, involving neurological mechanisms in the 'pleasure pathway' of the medial forebrain bundle and associated structures, and with dopamine as the main neurotransmitter. Drug abuse is an unpredictable phenomenon which involves biochemical, genetic, neurochemical, social, environmental, psychological and economic factors. There are also intrinsic properties of the drug that may influence its potential for abuse. These include:

- Lipid solubility: drugs with high lipid solubility rapidly achieve therapeutic concentrations within the central nervous system.
- Water solubility: water-soluble drugs are more easily prepared for injection.
- Volatility: volatile drugs can be inhaled in vapour form.
- Heat stability: heat-stable drugs can be inhaled in smoke.

The various interractions between the drug and the individual can be considered in respect of two commonly used drugs: alcohol and cocaine. Alcohol is a freely available drug for which the genetic predisposition to addictive behaviour is important. Cocaine is less accessible but has a high inherent addictive potential. Genetic make-up does not protect the casual user from a risk of addiction.

The extent to which the opioid drugs used in clinical practice have the potential for unmasking addictive behaviour is unclear. There are many observational studies that support the idea of patients maintained on long-term opioids for considerable lengths of time without evidence of addictive behaviour. It should be remembered, however, that there exist in society a proportion of patients who have at some time abused drugs and whose behaviour with treatment will need careful monitoring. There is also the real threat of violence against patients known to have supplies of opioids, and a risk that such drugs will be used by others than those for whom they were intended.

Practical management of opioids in chronic pain

The management of chronic pain of non-malignant origin with opioids remains controversial, not least because of the ethical difficulties involved in conducting proper randomized controlled trials in opioid-naïve patients with chronic pain. The use of drugs with a 'low ceiling' effect such as codeine or a partial agonist such as buprenorphine may protect the prescriber against fears of producing dependency or addictive behaviour, but may not be the most appropriate for the patient or the condition. The claim that tramadol does not have intrinsic 'addictive' properties is based on observations of opioid preferences in addicts – it is not widely used by them. This does not necessarily mean that it has intrinsic safety in pain patients. It is more appropriate that a decision is made that the pain is likely or not likely to respond to opioids, that other issues in respect of distress or illness behaviour are dealt with and a decision is made early to use or not to use this class of drugs than it is to rely on a theoretical ceiling effect to avoid the complications of dependency. The route and timing of administration is important. Avoidance of high peak drug levels in the brain mandates the use of slow-release preparations administered by the oral or transdermal route, rather than 'as required' doses by the intramuscular or buccal route. Similarly, it is important to recognize that if there is a need for a strong opioid, there is a continuing requirement. The use of these drugs presupposes an incurable nociceptive cause and a brain whose receptors will have become used to the presence of drug. There is little logic in the occasional use of opioid for chronically painful conditions, unless the natural history of the underlying condition is characterized by fluctuations in nociceptive stimulus, as in for example the patient with recurrent urinary tract stone formation or sickle cell disease.

Given that it may be appropriate for patients with chronic pain and a normal life expectancy to receive opioids, it is worth considering how the process is monitored. A careful lookout has to be made for behaviour that is suspicious of wrong usage. The term pseudoaddiction is used to describe the behaviour of the pain sufferer who achieves some, but suboptimal, pain relief from opioids and requests more. Requests for increases in dose may be plausible or less so: the way in which these requests are phrased may indicate whether or not the patient is appropriately using the drug. A preference for one particular type or brand of opioid analgesic may be justifiable, as may be the practice of hoarding of the drug to use when the pain is severe. However, bizarre explanations of the fate of drugs which were prescribed but never used – 'the dog ate it' or 'I left it on the train' – should raise suspicions of wrong usage.

The acceptability and availability of opioids varies greatly between countries and reflects the importance that fear of wrong use is held. This fear may be sanctioned by the state, whose doctors may be viewed with suspicion if they prescribe opioids. Morphine may carry with it the stigma of addiction or terminal illness, and may not be used by the patient who needs it. Opioids such as fentanyl and oxycodone may not be recognized as morphine-like substances by the public, and preferences for one particular drug may have less to do with quality of pain relief afforded by the drug than the beliefs and fears of the patient.

Practical aspects of opioid use: patient selection, prescribing and monitoring

Opioids are not effective in every patient with pain, although the concept that a pain is either responsive or non-responsive to opioids is an oversimplification. Some neuropathic pain, generally considered to be non-responsive, may respond, and a trial may be worthwhile. Assessment should consider the underlying cause of the pain, the response to previous simple analgesics and adjuvant agents if used. It is important to recognize the patient with a potential for misuse. It is important to identify a history of drug or alcohol abuse, psychiatric comorbidity and chaotic social circumstances. If opioid therapy is to be considered in these patients, appropriate help should be sought from colleagues with expertise in these areas.

Patients and health care professionals should agree a treatment plan prior to starting opioid therapy. Opioids should be considered to be only one aspect of an overall rehabilitative strategy. The primary outcome should be pain relief,

Patient ID: ....

SECTION 1 – complete for all patients on opiates
Diagnosis ....
Drug name ....
Dose regimen prescribed ....

SECTION 2 – complete for patients newly started on opiates
Has the patient tried adjuvants? (which) ....
Response to adjuvants   **Failed/Intolerant/Partial relief**

....
....

Ideas/Concerns/Expectations **from the patient** (e.g. Dependence/Tolerance/Drug of misuse)
Ideas/Concerns/Expectations **from the doctor**

....
....

Outcome goals explained	**Yes/No**
Treatment plan explained	**Yes/No**
Side effects discussed	**Yes/No**
Driving advice given	**Yes/No**
Follow up appointment (interval)	.... weeks
Patient information leaflet	**Yes/No**

SECTION 3 – complete for patients on follow up (on opiates)
If recorded, circle appropriate response:
Pain relief

much worse	*somewhat worse*	*no different*	*somewhat better*	*much better*

Physical

much worse	*somewhat worse*	*no different*	*somewhat better*	*much better*

Psychological

much worse	*somewhat worse*	*no different*	*somewhat better*	*much better*

Social function

much worse	*somewhat worse*	*no different*	*somewhat better*	*much better*

Current dose ....

Side effects
Nausea/Pruritis/Somnolence/Constipation/Cognitive/Sweating/Nil
....
....

Ideas/Concerns/Expectations **from the patient** (e.g. Dependence/Tolerance/Drug of misuse)
....
....

Ideas/Concerns/Expectations **from the doctor** (e.g. Is the pain opiate
responsive/tolerance/problem drug use, etc.)
....
....

Opioid switching ⇒ **Yes/No** *If YES, switched to* ....

Figure 1. Example of documentation used to monitor a patient on chronic opioid therapy. © RD Makin.

accompanied by improvements in physical, psychological and social function. Emphasis should be given to agreeing desirable treatment goals, and the time course over which these goals should be attained. Functional goals should be realistic and in context: for instance, in an otherwise fit patient return to work may be important, whereas for a disabled or elderly patient the ability to sit comfortably may be a valuable goal.

A contract agreed at the start of treatment sets out the patient's rights and responsibilities and may help to emphasize the importance of patient involvement and the consequences of non-compliance with the agreed treatment plan, including the circumstances which lead to discontinuation of treatment. Nurse practitioners with extended prescribing skills may assist with monitoring and maintaining opioid therapy within the agreed treatment plan, though the use of a single, identifiable doctor, responsible for prescribing may help to identify problem use if it occurs.

The use of sustained-release opioids administered at regular intervals is logical and to be recommended. In contrast, short-acting opioid preparations may predispose to tolerance and dependence and should not be used for the routine management of chronic non-cancer pain. Their use may reinforce 'pill for pain' behaviour in which the rapid rise in plasma and brain levels leads to a state of transient well-being that has to be repeated as the plasma level drops. Pethidine is recognized as particularly unsuitable for chronic use because of these characteristics.

Drug doses should be increased at fixed intervals following an initial successful trial period, and titrated up to the optimum dose. The patient assessment is key to establishing the optimal dose which provides the best balance of pain relief, functional improvement and side effects.

Patients should be monitored closely during the dose titration; this should occur at least monthly. During this periodic review, assessment should be made of the patient's self-report of pain, changes in physical and psychosocial function, onset of side effects and evidence of problem drug use or behaviour. The author's assessment chart used for this purpose is reproduced in Figure 1.

Further reading

Allan L, Hays H, Jensen N-H, et al. Randomised crossover trial of transdermal fentanyl and sustained release oral morphine for treating chronic non-cancer pain. British Medical Journal 2001; 322: 1154–8.

Hymes JA. Chemical dependency issues in patients with low back pain. Seminars in Spine Surgery 1996; 8(3): 202–7.

Portenoy RK. Opioid tolerance and responsiveness: research findings and clinical observations. In: Gebbart GF, Hammond DL, Jensen TS, eds. Proceedings of the 7th World Congress on Pain, Progress in Pain Research and Management, Vol. 2. Seattle: IASP Press, 1994; pp. 595–620.

Related topic of interest

Cancer pain – drugs (p. 50).

THERAPY – PARACETAMOL

Paracetamol (acetaminophen) is a *p*-aminophenol derivative. It was discovered in Germany in the late 19th century, but did not become widely used until the 1960s. It has analgesic and antipyretic, but not anti-inflammatory properties. Its mechanism of action remains unknown. Recent evidence suggests that it has an inhibitory effect on a specific cyclo-oxygenase 3 (COX 3) enzyme in the central nervous system but it is unclear how this relates to its clinical properties.

With oral usage, it is absorbed almost completely from the small bowel with about 20% first-pass metabolism, due to sulphation in the gut wall. Binding to plasma proteins is 20–50%. Peak plasma concentration occurs at about 1 hour, and plasma $t_{1/2}$ is 2–3 hours.

Use and efficacy

In the UK there is little variation in its adult dosage, 1 g four times a day by month, although in the USA the common starting dose is 650 mg four times a day, and doses up to 1.5 g four times a day are occasionally used. It is available as a suppository formulation, commonly used in the perioperative period, and as two intravenous products: propacetamol, a prodrug with a standard adult dose of 2 g, and more recently, a solution of paracetamol itself, with a standard adult dose of 1 g, both given four times a day. Only the latter formulation has a UK licence.

The oral formulation is often marketed in combination with moderate opioids (e.g. codeine, dihydrocodeine, tramadol), and is often used with stronger opioids (e.g. morphine). There is good evidence that its use in this way helps to reduce the opioid dose required, and consequently opioid side effects such as nausea, pruritus and constipation.

It is commonly given with nonsteroidal anti-inflammatory drugs (NSAIDs), although evidence to prove its efficacy in this way is less compelling.

Systematic reviews from meta-analysis for acute moderate to severe pain show the number needed to treat (NNT) (50% pain relief) for 1 g alone is 3.8 (3.4–4.4), for paracetamol 1 g plus codeine 60 mg is 2.2 (1.7–3.9) and for paracetamol plus tramadol is around 2–3 depending on the formulation used.

Both the codeine and tramadol studies showed significant minor morbidity.

Unwanted effects

At normal dosage, paracetamol has surprisingly few side effects. There is no gastric irritation, or bleeding abnormalities, as seen with the NSAIDs, or central nervous system (CNS) disturbance, as seen with opioids. There are occasional reports of rashes and blood disorders.

Liver. Paracetamol is metabolized in the liver, using glucuronide and sulphate conjugation. These metabolites are excreted via the kidneys. A small amount is normally metabolized into NAPQI (*N*-acetyl-*p*-benzoquinone imine). This has potentially hepatotoxic properties but is inactivated with a sulphydryl/thiolol

(–SH) donor, usually glutathione. In overdosage (>10–15 g), the –SH donors are rapidly depleted, and levels of NAPQI rise, leading to liver failure and death. The use of i.v. *N*-acetylcysteine and oral methionine, both –SH donors, within 12 hours is the therapy of choice.

Kidney. Phenacetin (a prodrug) and acetanilide are recognized for causing renal papillary necrosis and chronic interstitial nephritis when used chronically. It is uncertain whether paracetamol has this effect and it is more commonly seen with NSAIDs. There is usually some recovery on the withdrawal of the drug.

INDEX

Page numbers in *italics* indicate figures or tables.

Koller, Carl 118

laminectomy 42, 43, 103
lamotrigine 207
laparoscopy, diagnostic 168
laser therapy
  disc prolapse 42
  low level (LLLT) 149–50, 167
lateral cutaneous nerve of thigh, lesioning 162
learning difficulty 195
legal aspects 4
leg pain
  back pain with 36, 37, 44
  crossed 24
  epidural steroid injections 31
  physical examination 24, 26
  spinal cord stimulation 44, 155
  see also radicular pain; sciatica
levobupivacaine 120
L'Hermitte's sign 92, 93
lidocaine 205
  intranasal 205
  intravenous 205
    in burns 49
  subcutaneous, in cancer pain 55
  topical 121, 205
    in burns 49
    in post-herpetic neuralgia 133, 205
ligamentous back pain 36
limb pain
  phantom 106, 222
  physical examination 26
  see also brachialgia; leg pain
local anaesthetic blocks 104–8, 121–2
  in complex regional pain syndrome 65, 66
  diagnostic *see* nerve blocks, diagnostic
  long-term 122
  in neuralgias and peripheral neuropathies
    129–30
  for neuromata 142
  in post-herpetic neuralgia 133
  pre-emptive analgesia 106, 122–3
  in stroke patients 200
  sympathetic system 119–20, 124, 126, 202
  technique 106–8
  see also nerve blocks
local anaesthetics 118–23
  central neuraxial blockade 122–3
  clinical use 121–2
  history 118
  infiltration 121
  pharmacology 118–20
  topical *see* topical anaesthesia
  toxicity 120–1
locus of control 183

loin pain
  haematuria and 170–1
  recurrent, in pregnancy 177–8
loperamide 90
lorazepam, in burns 49
low back pain
  acute and chronic, management 37–8
  antidepressants 209
  assessment 34
  facet syndrome 37
  ligamentous 36
  lumbar segmental dysfunction 37
  medical management 34–9
  in multiple sclerosis 92, 93–4
  nerve root involvement 35
  non-specific (idiopathic) 34, 35–6
  from sacroiliac joints 37
  serious or systemic disease (red flags) 34–5
  surgery 43–4
  from vertebral body 37
  see also back pain
low-level laser therapy (LLLT) 149–50, 167
lumbar disc disease (prolapse) 40–2
  central 41, 42
  far lateral 35, 41
  investigations 41
  nerve root involvement 35, 40
  treatment 31, 41–2
  'typical' 40
lumbar segmental dysfunction 37
lumbar spinal stenosis 42–3
lumbar spine, physical examination 23–5
lumbar sympathetic chain block 125–6
  adverse effects 64, 126
  in complex regional pain syndrome 64
  technique 31, 125–6
lung carcinoma 113, 164
lung disease, chronic 59
lung pathology, chest pain 59
lymphoedema 144

magnetic resonance imaging (MRI)
  in back pain 36, 41, 43
  in cervical disc disease 102
  functional (fMRI) 8, 9, 44, 80, 159, 160, 189
  in trigeminal neuralgia 135, 138–9
malingering 4, 182
manipulation under anaesthesia, frozen
  shoulder 98
maxillo-facial surgeons 73
medical history, past 21
medicolegal reporting 4
medroxyprogesterone acetate 169, 170
memantine 223
meningiomas, spinal 45

sympathetically maintained pain (SMP) 129,
202–4
diagnosis 202–3
mechanisms 202
treatment 203–4
sympathetic blockade 124–7, 202
in cancer pain 111, 112
in chronic refractory angina 57
clinical indications 126
in complex regional pain syndrome 63–5, 66
diagnostic 124, 129, 202–3
intravenous regional 63–4, 126, 202–3
local anaesthetics 119–20, 124, 126, 202
in neuralgias and peripheral neuropathies
129
in scar pain 142–3
techniques 124–6
in vulval pain 173
sympathetic communicating ramus 28
destructive techniques 31
sympathetic ganglion block
in complex regional pain syndrome 64–5
see also stellate ganglion block
sympathetic nervous system 202–4
in complex regional pain syndrome 61
pelvic innervation 168–9
sympathomimetic drugs 203
symphysis pubis diastasis pain 177
symptom(s)
amplification 184
expectation 183
history taking 20–1
syndrome X 58
syrinx 46, 196, 197
systematic reviews 15–16

temporal arteritis 79, 96
temporomandibular joint (TMJ)
disease 73–4
dysfunction 73–4
internal derangement 73, 74
tender points, fibromyalgia 95–6
tendinopathy, subacute and chronic 150
TENS see transcutaneous electrical nerve
stimulation
tension headache 69, 84–5
tetracaine 121
9-tetrahydrocannabinol (δ9-THC) 217–18
thalamic pain 199
therapy, pain
in children 190, 191–2
history of previous 21
in pregnancy 174–6
see also drug treatment; non-
pharmacological interventions

thoracic back pain, examination 24
thoracic disc disease 44–5
thoracic paravertebral chain blocks 125
thoracic paravertebral injection 125
thoracic sympathetic blockade 125
in chronic refractory angina 57
thoracotomy, chronic pain after 143
tizanidine 203
tolerance, opioid 53, 226
topical anaesthesia 121
in post-herpetic neuralgia 133
topical treatments
for neuralgia/peripheral neuropathy 130
see also capsaicin; fentanyl, transdermal;
transcutaneous electrical nerve
stimulation
topiramate 207
in complex regional pain syndrome 66
in multiple sclerosis 93
tramadol 225
for cancer pain 51–2
in chronic pain 227
number needed to treat 17
paracetamol combination 231
transcutaneous electrical nerve stimulation
(TENS) 146–7
in chronic refractory angina 57
limitations 147
in multiple sclerosis 93
in neuralgia/peripheral neuropathy 130
in osteoarthritis 167
in post-herpetic neuralgia 133
in pregnancy 174
in spinal cord injury 197–8
technique of use 147
in temporomandibular joint dysfunction 74
uses 146
triamcinolone injections 98, 175
tricyclic antidepressants 209–10
in central post-stroke pain 200
in chronic post-surgical pain 144
in complex regional pain syndrome 66
in multiple sclerosis 93
in neuralgia/peripheral neuropathy 130
in post-herpetic neuralgia 132
in spinal cord injury 198
vulval pain 172–3
trigeminal autonomic cephalgias 76, 82–4
trigeminal (Gasserian) ganglion, lesioning
136–7, 139, 162
trigeminal nerve
microvascular decompression (MVD) 134,
137–9
nerve blocks via foramen ovale 136–7
peripheral neurolytic lesions 136